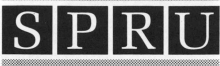

SOCIAL POLICY RESEARCH UNIT

Different Types of Care,
Different Types of Carer:

EVIDENCE FROM
THE GENERAL HOUSEHOLD SURVEY

Gillian Parker and
Dot Lawton

London: HMSO

ISBN 0 11 701783 3

This discussion paper is based on work funded by the Department of Health
but the opinions expressed are those of the authors alone.

SPRU Editorial Group

Sally Baldwin
Lorna Foster
Roy Sainsbury
Patricia Thornton
Peter Whiteford

Editor for this paper: Sally Baldwin

British Library Cataloguing in Publication Data

A catalogue record for this book is available from the British Library.

Acknowledgements

This book draws on research commissioned by the Department of Health and carried out at the Social Policy Research Unit at the University of York.

Material from the General Household Survey was made available through the Office of Population Censuses and Surveys (OPCS) and the ESRC Data Archive has been used by permission of the Controller of HSMSO. This further analysis and the interpretation of it are entirely the responsibility of the authors.

Contents

List of tables and figures

Counting carers

Introduction

Recent years have seen a growing recognition in Britain of the importance of 'informal care': the support and assistance provided on an informal basis to disabled and older people living in the community, usually by family members and close friends. In 1985 a review of existing research on informal care had to rely heavily on secondary sources (Parker, 1985); now it is becoming increasingly difficult to keep up with the wealth of research and writing on informal care and carers (Parker, 1990a and Twigg, 1992).

Much of this research and writing, however, has been based on relatively small-scale, often qualitative, approaches, with samples selected in such a way that extrapolation to the population of carers as a whole has been difficult. Some commentators tried to estimate numbers by extrapolating either from national surveys of disability or from small-scale research on informal care (Equal Opportunities Commission, 1982; Parker, 1985). By definition, these exercises could produce little more than 'guestimates'.

In the early 1980s the Department of Health and Social Security, responding to the increased interest in informal care, requested the Office of Population Censuses and Surveys (OPCS) to include a series of questions about this topic in its continuous national survey of adults in private households in Great Britain – the General Household Survey (GHS). These questions were included in the 1985 survey, a report was published in mid-1988 (Green, 1988), and the data became available for secondary analysis in early 1989 (Office of Population Censuses and Surveys, 1989).

All adults who were interviewed in the survey were asked whether they looked after or gave special help to anyone 'sick, handicapped, or elderly' living in the same household, or if they provided 'some regular service or help' to anyone 'sick, handicapped, or elderly' who lived in a different household.

The published report showed that one adult in seven (14 per cent) in Great Britain was providing informal care and that one in five households (19 per cent) contained a carer (Green, 1988). When applied to the whole population of Great Britain this suggested that there were approximately six million carers, 2.5 million men and 3.5 million women. However, it was clear that not all of those identified were providing the intensive and potentially difficult sort of care that previous small-scale research had mostly been concerned with. Indeed, the report itself often concentrated on those caring for 20 hours or more (24 per cent of the total).

It seemed highly likely, on the evidence of previous research, that the type and intensity of care provided, and who it was provided for, would influence the experience of caring in a number of important ways. The initial analysis of the data, presented in the report, did not allow these issues to be pursued fully.

Secondary analysis, by contrast, has been able to pull apart the global picture of informal caring produced by the survey. Several researchers have been involved in programmes of further analysis but, inevitably, each has pursued slightly different questions in somewhat different ways. Arber and Ginn (1990, 1991 and 1992) have concerned themselves predominantly with those who support older people, and have mostly distinguished between carers on the basis of whether or not they are looking after someone in the same household. Evandrou (1990) has used the carer's level of responsibility for the cared-for person as a major distinguishing characteristic. The analysis reported in this paper is based on *all* carers and develops a new approach by using patterns of caring *activity* to distinguish between different types of carers. The programme of analysis on which this work was based was commissioned by the Department of Health.

The policy context

The delivery of health and social care to people with physical or mental impairments or with general frailty associated with old age is currently a major social policy issue in Britain. The National Health Service and Community Care Act (1990) is set to revolutionise, particularly, social care provision. An emphasis on needs-led (rather than service-led) assessment, care management, the targeting of resources, the development of mixed economies of care, and the transfer of substantial sums of money from the Department of Social Security to local authority social services departments, all throw into question accepted and existing patterns of service provision and receipt.

Informal carers play a key role in maintaining disabled and older people in the community. The vast majority of disabled and older people live in private households, and the majority of these are supported and assisted by their family, friends and neighbours (Parker, 1990a). Despite this, informal carers occupy an ambiguous position in relation both to policy and to the social care system (Twigg, 1989; Baldwin and Parker, 1989). At the same time, they are peripheral to the social care system as Twigg (1989) argues, and yet essential to its functioning. Until very recently, policy documents rarely acknowledged that informal carers might have needs of their own; rather they were seen as the natural means by which disabled and older people should continue to be supported in the community:

> the primary sources of support and care for elderly people are informal and voluntary ... It is the role of public authorities to sustain and, where necessary, develop – but never to displace – such support and care. Care *in* the community must increasingly mean care *by* the community. (Cmnd 8173, 1981 para 1.9, original emphasis)

Carers thus occupied a 'strange Alice-in-Wonderland place where they [were] the main providers of community care but never the subjects of policy that [dealt] with the provision of care' (Baldwin and Parker, 1989, p. 157).[1]

More recently, the growth of research on informal care and the development of a very active carers' lobby has meant that informal carers have had to be incorporated into policy discussion. The Griffiths report (1988) has references throughout to the need to support informal carers, to provide them with information, to consult them as part of joint planning processes, and generally about 'how they can be helped with their onerous responsibilities' (Griffiths, 1988, para. 4.13). Further, those who plan care are encouraged to take into account the views and wishes of informal carers, as well as those of the person they assist.

The White Paper, 'Caring for People', asserts that 'a key responsibility of statutory service providers should be to do all they can

---

[1] Except in relation to social security policy where carers' needs were recognised in the 1974 White Paper, 'Social Security Provision for Chronically Sick and Disabled People'. This led to the introduction of a new benefit, the Invalid Care Allowance (ICA) in 1975.

to assist and support carers' (Department of Health, Cm 849, 1989, para. 2.2). Similarly, policy and practice guidance following from the passing of the NHS and Community Care Act 1990 underline the role of informal carers. The practice guidance, for example, states that carers' contributions should be 'formally recognised' in new care management and assessment procedures, and that, where necessary, carers 'should be offered a separate assessment of their own needs' (SSI/SWSG, 1991, para. 39, summary).

However, debate continues about whether the inclusion of these statements in policy documents will mean any change for the majority of carers. The benefits of care management processes for informal carers remain contested (Parker, 1990b) while anxieties about funding levels for community care raise questions about the extent to which informal carers will have any of their current responsibilities lightened (King's Fund Centre, 1992).

The picture for informal carers, then, is mixed. On the one hand they are, for the first time, acknowledged as the major providers of 'community care'; on the other hand, it remains difficult to see how much of existing and new resources will be given over to supporting or relieving them.

Whatever the outcome of the new community care arrangements the profile of informal carers and caring has been raised and cannot be ignored. Service planners and providers, whether in social services or the health service, whether in the statutory or independent sectors, need to *know* about carers – who they are, whom they help and support, what they do, and the impact that caring has on their lives. Detailed analysis of the GHS data is one way to provide that information.

Care, caring or carers: problems of definition

Although the idea of 'care' is one most people would claim to understand, it is one many would have difficulty in defining. As Bulmer has said:

> The meaning of care is intuitively fairly obvious, referring to the provision of help, support and protection for vulnerable and dependent members of society. It is not often clear, however, what types of help, support and protection are meant when the term is used. (Bulmer, 1987, p.19)

In his influential article in 1981, Roy Parker made the distinction between 'care' which is concern about people and care which is more properly thought of as 'tending'. The first 'may find expression in a charitable donation, in lobbying, in prayer or in feelings of anxiety, sadness or pleasure at what happens to others' while the second 'describes the actual work of looking after those who, temporarily or permanently, cannot do so for themselves' (Parker, 1981, p.17). It is with the second type of care that this paper is primarily concerned although, as should become evident, the two types are not entirely distinct, either conceptually or practically.

A number of commentators and researchers in this field have attempted to define or distinguish between different sorts of caring activity or behaviour – both concern and tending – in order to provide a basis for understanding neighbouring, friendship, 'informal' care, 'community care' and related concepts. For the purposes of this paper it is the tending end of the spectrum that is of major interest.

The basis for the definition even of tending activity has varied substantially between researchers and commentators, but the first step, for most, has been to describe or name the tasks that are carried out. Beyond this, however, the ways in which the named tasks are categorized differ.

Elements of timing, frequency, urgency, complexity, and how long the tasks take, have been used singly or in combination, and in different ways as a second step in imposing some order on the tasks. In most cases this order is either implicitly or explicitly hierarchical.

Characteristics of the context in which tasks are carried out are sometimes used as a third element when categorizing tending activity. Examples here include the nature and/or level of the cared-for person's impairment, whether or not the cared-for person's presence is essential to the task, and the level of responsibility the carer carries.

Finally, some categorizations try to incorporate elements which are less about practical tasks and more about the defined emotional 'work' of caring, such as 'nurturing', 'comforting' or 'supporting'.

It is not surprising, given the range of possible combinations within and between these different elements, that there is relatively little comparability between the categorizations used by different researchers and writers. Beyond a basic underlying agreement of what constitutes a personal care task and what a domestic or household task, it is difficult to find common ground between them.

As well as attempting to categorize what informal carers *do*, the literature also tries to categorize who informal carers *are*. The nature of the relationship between the carer and the cared-for person is, thus, the other major analytical break to be found in the literature on the provision of informal care. For example, there have been studies which have concentrated on parents caring for children with disabilities (Glendinning, 1983; Baldwin, 1985; Ayer and Alaszewski, 1984), on daughters caring for mothers (Lewis and Meredith, 1988), on spouses caring for a disabled husband or wife (Parker, 1993), and so on. Within these categories the sex and age of the carer, and sometimes the sex and age of the cared-for person, have also been important discriminating variables. Thus the fathers and mothers of disabled children, the sons and daughters of frail elderly people, husbands and wives, have been compared and contrasted.

Finally, there have been attempts to categorize informal carers in terms of why they care. Ungerson (1987), for example, has devised a typology of carers based on their motivations and on their position in the life-cycle.

In sum, then, the existing literature attempts to analyse the nature of informal caring using four dimensions: what is done, who does it, for whom, and why (Figure 1.1).

Figure 1.1   The dimensions of caring

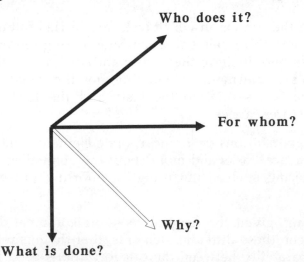

An essential first step in the secondary analysis of the 1985 GHS data reported here was an attempt to identify common criteria which previous writers had used to categorize caring activity and carers. We did not wish merely to impose our own categorization if some commonly applied or understood framework already existed. However, as is obvious from the brief review presented above, this was not the case.

Obviously, the GHS itself had imposed some framework on the data, both through pre-coding on the questionnaire and through post-coding for analysis. Information about carers covered their sex, their relationship to the cared-for person, the sex of the cared-for person, the nature of their disability and a host of other socio-economic data gathered routinely from GHS respondents. In addition, the caring activities were coded into eight main areas:

- help with personal care (e.g. dressing, bathing, toileting)

- physical help (e.g. with walking, getting in and out of bed)

- help with paperwork or financial matters

- other practical help (e.g. preparing meals, doing shopping, housework, household repairs)

- keeping the cared-for person company

- taking the cared-for person out

- giving medicine (includes giving injections or changing dressings)

- keeping an eye on the cared-for person to see he/she is all right

We could have used the characteristics of the carers, the characteristics of those being cared for, the nature of caring activities carried out, or some combination of these, as the basis for our analytical framework. For a variety of reasons we decided to use the tasks alone and to develop a typology of caring activity.

The main reason for this decision was to take a different approach from previous research which had categorized carers in terms of who they, or those they cared for, were and had then gone on to describe what they did. It seemed likely to us that what people do might be influenced by who they and the person they were helping were. To describe the full range of caring activity identified in the population it seemed important, in the first instance at least, to distance it from its social or relational context.

The second reason this approach was adopted was an attempt to question some of the sweeping generalisations that were being made, on the basis of GHS data, about the number of carers in the population. The figure of six million carers supporting highly dependent people in the community is in danger of becoming received wisdom. It was clear from an initial look at the GHS data that the level of involvement of some of those included in this six million was not substantial and could not, in any way, be seen as comparable to the level of involvement identified in earlier, small-scale studies of caring. A description and enumeration of different patterns or types of caring activity seemed an obvious place to start if more discriminating population estimates were to be attempted.

Thirdly, it seemed that an analysis of caring activity was a more useful approach when looking for recommendations for policy development or revised forms of practice in order to support carers. Given the existing shape of service provision, and the current emphasis on needs-led provision, it seemed more helpful to think about providing support on the basis of what carers *do* rather than on the basis of who they *are*. This is not to deny that the relationship between the carer and the cared-for person may influence both perceived need for support and the way in which that support might best be delivered (Twigg and Atkin, 1993). Rather it acknowledges that knowing what carers do has a clear, 'service-shaped', relevance while knowing only who they are can imply a whole range of different levels of involvement and, therefore, needs for support.

Once the decision was made to use caring tasks as the basis of the categorization the next decision was how we should impose a framework over and above that already implied by the GHS classification of tasks. We have already seen that the literature did not offer us a ready guide but we could have used elements of other researchers' categorizations as a starting point. However, we decided to let the data speak for themselves. We already knew that there was overlap between different caring tasks – respondents had been able to identify any or all of the activities they carried out. We therefore decided to proceed on the assumption that we might find some systematic overlapping which would allow us to say confidently that different *patterns* of caring activity were discernible in the community at large. In Chapter Two we describe how these different patterns were identified, while in Chapter Three we use the patterns of caring activity to explore the consequences of caring. In Chapters Four and Five we examine service receipt among those with informal carers and attempt to account for the variations found. In the final chapter we draw conclusions from our analysis about the continuing need to collect data on carers.

Different types of caring

Developing the typology

The first step in developing a typology of caring activity was to look at how different caring 'tasks' were associated with one another.

The analysis was based on the number of people being helped, rather than the number of carers. This was because 504 carers were recorded as looking after more than one person. To have used the number of carers as the base would have clouded the picture of the way in which caring tasks go together. For example, a carer helping two people might have provided personal, physical and practical help to one, but have taken the other one out and kept an eye on him/her. These are different patterns of caring responsibility but if the carer is used as the basis of analysis and the caring tasks amalgamated the pattern is lost (see Appendix 1 for further discussion).

Three thousand and sixty-one cared-for people were identified. For 29 of these no information was recorded on the nature of help that they received. The following analysis is thus based on 3,032 'instances' of caring.

As Table 2.1 shows, certain types of task were much more common than others. It is also obvious that there must have been substantial overlap in the tasks being carried out. The next step in developing the typology was to examine this overlap.

First, it was clear that there was more overlap between some tasks than between others. For example, on 90 per cent of occasions when help was given with medicines, practical help was also provided. By contrast, in only 22 per cent of cases where practical help was provided was personal or physical help also given.

Secondly, involvement in some tasks was likely to imply a high level of involvement in the whole range of tasks. When personal or physical help was provided there was a high level (50 per cent or more) of involvement in all other types of caring. By contrast, when practical help was being given there was relatively high involvement in only two other caring tasks, keeping company and keeping an eye on.

Table 2.1   Incidence of caring tasks

Type of caring task	N	%*
Personal care	654	22
Physical care	612	20
Paperwork	1,173	39
Practical	2,474	82
Keeping company	1,939	64
Taking out	1,441	48
Giving medicine	603	20
Keeping an eye on	2,148	71
Base (100%)	3,032	

* sums to more than 100% because categories are not mutually exclusive

These patterns of overlap, coupled with the strength of association between the various caring tasks (see Table 2.2), gave some indication of those variables which might be grouped together in order to start constructing a typology.

Clustering the caring tasks

The two-way comparison of caring tasks was a useful start in discerning patterns among them. However, it was obvious, even from visual inspection of the data, that three or more tasks could be inter-related. For example, personal care was strongly associated with physical care and giving medicine, while physical care was of itself strongly associated with giving medicine.

In order to explore the inter-relationships among tasks, cluster analysis was used.[2] The clustering procedure was used experimentally and iteratively to generate categories which appeared to be relatively distinct. Obviously it was not possible to develop

[2] This is a statistical procedure which allows objects (cases) to be grouped according to their occurrence within cases. Several measures and methods are available which are used to group the cases or variables. In this case, lambda – a measure suitable for use with binary data – and within groups average linking were used (Aldenderfer and Blashfield, 1984).

Table 2.2 Degrees of association (contingency co-efficient*) between pairs of caring tasks

	Personal	Physical	Paperwork	Practical	Keeping company	Taking out	Giving medicine	Keeping an eye on
Personal	–	0.43	0.16	0.04	0.13	0.14	0.39	0.15
Physical		–	0.15	0.08	0.15	0.18	0.38	0.16
Paperwork			–	0.11	0.19	0.22	0.21	0.22
Practical				–	0.03**	0.01**	0.11	0.05
Keeping company					–	0.18	0.16	0.26
Taking out						–	0.13	0.16
Giving medicine							–	0.21
Keeping an eye on								–

* Maximum value of C (contingency coefficient) for 2 x 2 table is 0.71

** Not significant

a typology with completely watertight categories, particularly as many of the tasks were strongly associated. However, the final version of the typology was arrived at when it seemed that as much distance or distinction as possible had been made between different patterns.

The six mutually exclusive categories arrived at by this process are as follows:

● personal *and* physical care

● personal *not* physical care

● physical *not* personal care

● other practical help

● practical help only

● other help

A caring relationship fell into the first category if the carer provided personal care and physical help regardless of whether any other type of help was given. A caring relationship fell into the second category when personal care was provided but physical help was not, again regardless of the provision of other types of help.

Conversely, the third category contained relationships where physical help was given but not personal care. The remaining categories included only relationships where neither personal care nor physical help was given. The fourth category covered practical help plus any combination of help with paperwork, keeping company, taking out or keeping an eye on. In the fifth category practical help alone was given. The final category covered any combination of help with paperwork, keeping company, taking out, giving medicine or keeping an eye on.

Table 2.3   Categories of caring

Category	%
1. Personal *and* physical care	12
2. Personal *not* physical care	9
3. Physical *not* personal care	8
4. Other practical help	50
5. Practical help only	8
6. Other help	14
Base (100%)	3,032

Testing the typology

Having developed a typology based only on the relationships between caring tasks, the next stage was to test how well, if at all, it distinguished between different types of carers, cared-for people and caring relationships – between women and men, between different kin relationships, between younger and older carers, and so on.

Cross-tabulation between the caring typology and a range of other variables revealed that the typology did distinguish well between different sorts of carers and cared-for people. The variables used to test the typology were: an index of involvement in caring; sex of the carer; sex of the cared-for person; age of the carer; age of the cared-for person; relationship of the cared-for person to the carer; the nature of the cared-for person's impairment or illness; the number of hours per week for which care was provided; whether or not the cared-for person lived in the same household as the carer; and the carer's level of responsibility for the cared-for person.[3] There were significant differences in the distribution of each of these variables between different categories in the typology. However, some of these differences were more substantial than others.[4]

Overall involvement in caring tasks

The typology was highly related to the number of tasks carers were involved in. The average number of tasks involved in each instance of caring is, of course, determined by the category to which it is assigned. *Personal and physical care*,[5] for example, *could* involve eight caring tasks while *other practical*[5] could only ever involve a maximum of six tasks. However, if the average number of tasks carried out in each category is divided by the

---

[3] Readers interested in a detailed account of the way in which the typology was tested, including all relevant tables and statistical tests, are referred to the original working paper (Parker and Lawton, 1990a).

[4] Two measures were used to indicate, first, the strength of association between the caring typology and the variable in question and, secondly, the degree to which particular caring categories contributed to this strength of association. The first measure was the contingency co-efficient (c) a non-parametric 'measure of the extent of association or relation between two sets of attributes' (Siegel, 1956). The second measure was the adjusted standardised residual. This indicates which cells of a cross-tabulation are contributing most to the association. Cells with adjusted, standardised residuals of 1.96 are generally regarded as contributing significantly to the association. All the general relationships between the caring typology and individual variables, and all the particular relationships between specified values of those variables which are referred to in this chapter, were 'significant' in terms of one or other of the two measures described.

[5] Caring categories in the text are referred to in italics.

theoretical maximum for that category, we can calculate a 'task index'. Here we can see that the typology distinguishes well between categories on this basis (Table 2.4).

Sex of the carer
One of the most surprising findings to emerge from the original GHS analysis (Green, 1988) was the extent to which men were involved in caring. Prior to this the literature on informal care had suggested that men were very rarely involved in providing care and that, when they were, this was in some sense aberrant (see, for example, Ungerson, 1987). By contrast the 1985 GHS found that 12 per cent of men in the population at large and 15 per cent of women identified themselves as carers.

Table 2.4   The task index in different categories of caring

Categories of caring	Mean task index*
1. Personal *and* physical care	0.83
2. Personal *not* physical care	0.64
3. Physical *not* personal care	0.67
4. Other practical help	0.57
5. Practical help only	n/a
6. Other help	0.42

* average number of tasks/maximum number of tasks possible

However, the 1985 GHS analysis also showed that female carers were more likely to be 'main' carers (that is, people who were sole carers or who spent more time than anyone else helping) and to be caring for 20 or more hours a week than were male carers. Further, men were substantially more likely to be caring for a woman (75 per cent) than women were to be caring for a man (33 per cent) but less likely to be providing personal care (Green, 1988, Tables 3.5 and 4.20).

Given these findings one might expect an adequate typology of caring to distinguish between men and women carers and this was the case with the typology developed here. Women were more likely to be involved in the first two types of care, which include providing personal care, while male carers were more likely to be providing *physical not personal care* and *practical help only*.

Sex of the cared-for person
The caring typology also distinguished significantly between those cases where the person being helped was male and those

where the person being helped was female although the strength of the relationship was not great.

Men were rather more likely than would be expected to be receiving *personal not physical care* while women were more likely to be receiving *practical help only.*

Age of the carer
Significant differences existed between different categories of caring and the ages of carers, but the association was not particularly strong. The oldest carers were over-represented in *personal and physical care*; some 22 per cent of carers in this category were aged 66 and over compared with 15 per cent of all carers.

Age of the cared-for person
The age of the cared-for person and the type of care being provided were strongly associated. However, the direction of the association was, perhaps, unexpected. Younger cared-for people, up to the age of 65, were over-represented in *personal and physical care* while the older cared-for people were over-represented in *practical help only* and *other practical help.* Obviously one would expect children to be more likely to be receiving personal care but it is somewhat surprising to find younger adults also over-represented here.

The finding that older people are more likely to be in receipt of practical, rather than personal, forms of care echoes findings from the 1980 and 1985 GHS which show that it is domestic tasks, rather than personal care tasks, which present many elderly people with problems. It also underlines recent research which demonstrates the extent to which elderly people strive to retain their independence (Wenger, 1984; Qureshi and Walker, 1989).

Relationship of cared-for person to carer
The nature of the relationship between the carer and the person being supported is another area which is believed to be important in determining the nature of care which might be provided. For example, much research has suggested that neighbours and distant kin are unlikely to be involved in providing more personal forms of care (Parker, 1990a). Did the typology of care differentiate between different relationships?

There was, indeed, a highly significant and strong association between the different categories of care and the relationship between the carer and the cared-for person. People helping those who were not close or blood relatives (parents-in-law, other relatives, friends and neighbours) were unlikely to be giving personal or physical types of care and were more likely to be giving practical forms of help. Those helping spouses and children (including adult children) were the groups most likely to be giving personal care, while those helping parents were most likely to give *physical not personal care* or *other practical help*.

Nature of impairment

Carers identified in the 1985 GHS were asked what was 'wrong' with the person they cared for and how this affected them – physically, mentally or both. The actual diagnosis was not coded but information on the type of impairment was. The final categorization also included 'old age' and 'other' types of impairment.

Quite clear patterns of association were evident between the type of caring and the type of impairment. People with both physical and mental impairments were over-represented in the first three categories of caring while people said to be suffering from 'just old age' were over-represented only in the last two categories. Again, these findings may challenge some of the received ideas about dependency in old age. They also demonstrate the importance of mental impairment in determining the provision of help with personal care.

The number of hours of help given

The 1985 GHS recorded a very wide range of involvement in caring, from people providing under two hours of help a week to those providing a hundred hours or more a week. Again, the caring typology distinguished clearly between these different levels of involvement.

There were very strong associations between categories involving personal care and levels of involvement of over 20 hours per week. For example, some 69 per cent of carers providing *personal and physical care* were caring for twenty or more hours per week. By contrast, types of help not involving personal or physical care were much more likely to be associated with lower levels of involvement. More than 7 out of 10 (72 per cent) of those providing *other practical help*, for example, were involved for fewer than 10 hours per week.

Living in the same household

Overall, only 25 per cent of carers lived in the same household as the person they were helping. However, there was wide variation across the caring categories. The first three categories of caring were highly associated with caring in the same household, particularly so within the *personal and physical care* category, where over two-thirds (68 per cent) of carers were in the same household as the person they helped. By contrast, the other three categories, particularly *other practical help* and *practical help only* were highly associated with care provision elsewhere. Almost nine out of ten people in the *other practical help* category lived in a different household from the person they helped.

Level of responsibility

The typology also distinguished well between carers with different levels of responsibility for the person being cared for. Overall, 29 per cent of carers said that they had sole responsibility but among those giving *personal and physical care* the proportion was 38 per cent. Some 70 per cent in this category were the sole or main carers. By contrast, only 52 per cent of those providing *other practical help* had sole or main responsibility.

Conclusion

The six types of caring, identified by clustering the caring task variables, distinguished well between carers on a number of important dimensions. While the six categories are not entirely 'watertight', detailed testing of the typology (Parker and Lawton, 1990) shows that they separate carers sufficiently well to suggest that they represent real 'types' of caring activity. A summary of the main features of carers in each category is given in Appendix 3.

As it was hoped it would, the caring typology provides a proxy measure for the degree of involvement in caring activity. This is a more refined measure than, say, just the number of hours of assistance carers provide each week; it is both a 'service-shaped' indicator *and* implies a number of other indicators of level of involvement – the average number of tasks carried out, caring in the same household, a high number of hours of care, older carers, physical *and* mental impairment of the person being helped, and sole or main responsibility. The caring categories, then, can be seen as summary indicators of the type and level of involvement of carers, with those giving *personal and physical care* being the most involved and those giving *other help* the least. In subsequent chapters, then, we are able both to explore the impact of level of involvement in caring and, where necessary, to control for it by using the typology.

By dividing up the large number of people identified in the 1985 GHS as 'carers', on the basis of the type of caring task they carry out, the caring typology should allow us to move to a more sophisticated understanding of the nature of informal caring activity.

On one hand, we have identified those people who are involved in substantial levels of caring activity, providing personal and physical care for long hours and over relatively long periods of time. These carers are often quite elderly themselves and are most likely to be caring for close relatives who live in the same household. On the other hand, we have identified very substantial groups of people involved in activities which might more accurately be termed 'informal helping'. They provide practical help to friends, neighbours and less close relatives, who do not live in the same household, for relatively few hours, but may do so over long periods of time. These 'helpers' seem to fall into two main sub-groups. First, there are those who are the only or main source of help for the other individual. Secondly, and more commonly, there are those who are part of a 'network' where others, presumably, take major responsibility.

These differences have obvious implications both for the type of services that might be required to support informal care in the community and for the numbers of carers that might need such support.

The 1985 GHS report (Green, 1988) suggested that around six million people in Great Britain were involved in providing care or help. Divided between the six categories developed in this paper this suggests that there are:

734,400 people providing *personal and physical care* (12 per cent of carers)

559,800 providing *personal not physical care* (9 per cent)

477,000 providing *physical not personal care* (8 per cent)

2,960,400 providing *other practical help* that is not personal or physical (50 per cent)

453,000 providing *practical help only* (8 per cent)

815,400 providing *other help* (14 per cent)

The total of 1.29 million people in the first two categories is very close to the estimates of the numbers of 'heavy end' carers produced before the 1985 GHS and also to estimates of the numbers of carers derived from the OPCS disability surveys (Parker, 1990a, p. 23).

The impact on people's lives of providing these different types of care and help, and the role that services play in supporting them are the main subjects of the next chapters.

The consequences of caring

Introduction

Previous research on informal care has suggested that the consequences of caring can include economic, physical, emotional and opportunity costs. Loss and restriction of employment, reduced income, increased expenditure, restricted family and social life, and physical and emotional strain have all been described. However, such effects may vary, depending on who is doing the caring and where. Further, while some effects may be the same across different sub-groups of carers or cared-for people, others, for example those relating to employment opportunities, may not (see Parker, 1990a for a review of the evidence).

With one or two notable exceptions the research which has described these effects has not compared the findings with the general population. Consequently, only a few effects can confidently be ascribed to caring and caring alone. These are: the financial effects of caring on the parents, particularly mothers, of children with severe disabilities (Baldwin, 1985; Smyth and Robus, 1989); the effects of caring on women's labour market participation (Joshi, 1987); and the raised levels of emotional strain experienced by carers compared to the population at large (Isaacs *et al.*, 1972; Bradshaw and Lawton, 1978; Levin *et al.*, 1983; Quine and Pahl, 1985).

The 1985 GHS appeared to offer an ideal opportunity to look at the consequences of caring in a systematic and controlled way; it was a large, nationally representative survey and distinguished between those with caring responsibilities and those without.

However, there are two major difficulties with interpretation of the GHS data. First, a straight comparison between carers and non-carers on a number of relevant variables – marital status, employment, income, health, for example – does, of course, reveal differences (see Appendix 3). The difficulty arises because, while some of these differences may well be the result of caring, others may be factors which determine whether or not an individual actually *becomes* a carer. Beyond those characteristics which are unchangeable – age and sex – we cannot be absolutely sure about the direction of the relationship between caring and other variables. For example, some people may become carers because their own health is not perfect and, therefore, they are less likely to be in the labour market. Or perhaps their own ill-health is an additional factor which predisposes them to leave paid work when they also have caring responsibilities. Alternatively, caring may actually have caused or exacerbated their ill-health. In the absence of any truly longitudinal data about the impact of informal care it is thus difficult to be absolutely sure about the direction of cause and effect.

The second major difficulty arises *because* carers are so different from non-carers. We know that carers, as a group, are very different from the population at large, regarding both sex and age. Women are more likely than men, and people over the age of 45 more likely than younger age groups, to be carers (Parker and Lawton, 1991). Given that sex and age influence a number of the variables on which we might wish to compare carers, a straight comparison becomes difficult.

A number of possibilities for dealing with these problems were explored in our analysis of the GHS. One was to use a quasi-longitudinal approach in an attempt to tease out cause and effect. For example, we could have compared the economic status of those who had been caring for different lengths of time. The difficulty here is that, by doing so, we would also have created age effects. Those caring for 20 or more years, say, are likely to be older than those who have been caring for five years.

To be useful, a quasi-longitudinal approach would also have to control for age. However, even if this were done, it is likely that cohort effects would also make interpretation difficult. For example, the relationship of 30 year old married women to the labour market twenty years ago would have been different from that of 30 year old married women today.

Another possible approach was to match carers with non-carers on a number of independent variables which seemed likely, from first principles, to influence the dependent variable of interest. For example, if we matched carers and non-carers by age and sex we might expect few differences between them in relation to marital status or health unless caring itself was truly related to the variable in question. This approach does not, of course, get us over the cause and effect problem. However, it is possible to make informed guesses about the direction of the relationship.

This matching approach is the one we adopted but the reader should bear in mind the reservations about interpretation given above. The way in which the two matched groups of 2,516 individuals were set up is described in Appendix 4. This appendix also describes the procedure which allowed us to compare people in different caring categories with matched non-carers, and to compare carers in the same and different households from the person they were helping with matched non-carers.

Marriage, households and caring

Marriage

One of the possible effects of becoming a carer, if it happens at a relatively early stage in life, is that it might alter the chances of the carer's marrying. The analysis presented here shows little evidence of an effect of this sort. The largest differences between the carers and matched non-carers were in the proportions who were *currently* married or widowed (Table 3.1). Despite the matching, carers were still more likely to be married than non-carers and less likely to be widowed, divorced or separated. Further, these patterns were more evident, and significant, among the female carers than among the males. However, while there was no overall evidence of caring being related to marital status some impact was evident amongst the most heavily involved carers (those providing both physical and personal care). Here, carers were very much more likely than non-carers to be single.

Table 3.1 **Marital status of carers and matched non-carers**

Marital status	Carer %	Non-carer %	All %
Married	74	71	73
Single	13	12	13
Widowed	7	10	9
Divorced	4	5	5
Separated	2	1	1
Base (100%)	2,516	2,516	5,032

$X^2 = 16.1$, df = 4, p< 0.01

The differences in marital status were also more evident among carers living in the same household as the person they helped (same household carers), where both married *and* single carers were significantly over-represented, than among different household carers.

These comparisons suggest two distinct patterns. First, there may be a tendency for carers to *become* carers because they are married. In a sense, they marry into potential responsibility, particularly for their own spouses but also for parents-in-law and other relatives. This pattern is evident regardless of sex but is a little stronger among females. By contrast, widowhood, divorce and separation reduce the likelihood of, at least, current caring responsibilities (we do not know whether these individuals had been carers in the past). Again, this is particularly the case for women.

The second effect was among those most heavily involved (*personal and physical care*). Here, carers were most likely to be single. We do not know definitively whether these carers remained single because they were carers or whether they became carers because they were single and, possibly, still living in their parents' home. Evidence from other studies, of both same household and different household caring, suggests that single (or divorced) offspring still living at home are more likely than their married siblings to become involved in caring for their parents (Glendinning, 1992; Qureshi and Walker, 1989). But even in these studies cause and effect are not clear.

Relationship to head of household

Carers have very different sorts of living arrangements from non-carers. Bearing in mind again that age and sex are already controlled for by the matching process, we find that carers are significantly less likely than non-carers to be the household head (46 per cent and 52 per cent respectively) and more likely to be classed as the child of the household head (eight per cent and five per cent respectively). This pattern was somewhat stronger among males than among females, but in both cases it was clear that carers were less likely to be a household head than non-carers.

This pattern was, as might be expected, particularly evident among same household carers. Seventeen per cent of same household carers were classed as the child of the household head compared to only four per cent of the matched, non-carer equivalents. This difference clearly echoes that found in relation to marital status where single carers were found to be over-represented among same household carers. Again, it was a pattern particularly evident among those most heavily involved in caring (*personal and physical care*).

Household size

As would be expected, carers were in larger households (inclusive of same household cared-for people) than non-carers. They were also much less likely to be in one-person households.

These differences may reflect a number of factors: disabled children do not leave home at the same time as their peers (Hirst, 1990); unmarried children stay in their parents' home longer in order to provide care, or have become carers because they are still at home when most of their peers have left; and joint households are formed when, particularly, elderly people become too frail to care for themselves. All, however, contribute to an 'extra person' effect.

However, the impact on household size was not spread evenly across all types of carers. Both male and female carers were less likely than non-carers to be in one-person households but it was only female carers who were significantly more likely to be in households of four or more people than their non-carer peers. This possibly reflects their greater involvement in caring for disabled, adult offspring.

Further, it is largely those most involved in caring who are in the bigger households. It is here, as well, that same household care is most likely to take place so this clearly reflects the 'extra-person' effect. The impact of being in a larger than expected household because of being a carer could be considerable – overcrowded accommodation and lower or higher per capita income spring to mind. These possibilities will be explored in more detail below.

Economic activity

It has been known for some years that providing care can have adverse effects on carers' labour market participation, particularly when the carers are women and are heavily involved (for example, Baldwin, 1985; Nissel and Bonnerjea, 1982). In its examination of labour market participation, the original 1985 GHS report concentrated only on carers devoting at least 20 hours a week to caring. This showed that 48 per cent of male carers and 40 per cent of female carers of working age had paid work while providing at least 20 hours of care. Women carers were far more likely than men (25 per cent compared to three per cent) to be in part-time work. The economic activity of individuals is, of course, related to age and sex, both separately and in combination. The impact of caring on economic activity, then, should be clear when these two variables have been controlled for.

The findings from the analysis presented here seem, initially at least, rather surprising. Tables 3.2 and 3.3 show that the effect of caring on employment is not, perhaps, as dramatic among the GHS respondents as might have been expected.

Table 3.2   Economic activity of carers and matched non-carers[*]

Marital status	Carer %	Non-carer %	All %
Full-time employment	44	52	48
Part-time employment	20	18	19
Seeking work	8	6	7
Permanently unable to work	4	3	3
Retired	3	3	3
Keeping house	18	16	17
Student	2	2	2
Other inactive	1	1	1
Base (100%)	1,887	1,871	3,758

$X^2 = 24.5$, df = 7 , p < 0.001
[*] all under pension age, 60 f, 65 m

Carers of working age *were* significantly less likely than their age/sex peers to be in full-time work but there was little difference in relation to part-time work. Where carers were overrepresented this was in relation to being permanently unable to work or seeking work. Carers were only slightly overrepresented among those keeping house.

The findings are even more surprising when we consider men and women separately (Table 3.3).

Although both male and female carers were less likely than their age peers to be in full-time paid work, this pattern was more strongly evident among men. Further, male carers were more likely than their peers to be classified as seeking work or keeping house. By contrast, female carers were more likely to be classified as permanently unable to work.

Table 3.3   Economic activity of carers and matched non-carers* by sex

Economic activity	Male[1]		Female[2]	
	Carer %	Non-carer %	Carer %	Non-carer %
Full-time employment	70	79	25	31
Part-time employment	3	1	32	30
Seeking work	12	9	5	4
Permanently unable to work	5	4	3	1
Retired	5	4	1	2
Keeping house	2	<1	30	28
Student	2	1	2	2
Other inactive	1	1	1	<1
Base (100%)	800	793	1,087	1,078

[1] $X^2 = 28.3$, df = 7, p < 0.001   [2] $X^2 = 17.3$, df = 7, p < 0.05
* all under pension age, 60f, 65m

Comparisons between carers in different caring categories showed that it was only among the most heavily burdened carers (*personal and physical care*) that *any* significant employment effects were evident. The difference in this group was, again, in the proportions in full-time work – 31 per cent of the carers compared with 47 per cent of the matched non-carers.

Differences were also evident when the location where caring took place was considered. Among the same household groups, only 42 per cent of carers were in full-time work compared to 52 per cent of non-carers. Part of the difference was made up by the higher proportion of carers who were classified as keeping house (21 per cent compared to 14 per cent of non-carers). A different pattern (and a weaker one) was evident among the different household groups. Again carers were less likely than non-carers to be in full-time paid work (45 per cent and 52 per cent respectively). However, this time the difference was made up by the higher proportions of carers in part-time work (22 per cent compared to 19 per cent) or who were seeking work (eight per cent compared to six per cent).

In sum, both female and male carers were less likely than matched non-carers to be in paid employment of any sort, but the difference was not so evident among women. This depressive effect was, however, present only among those providing both *personal and physical care* and only among those who cared for someone in the same household. While there was an overall negative relationship between caring and paid work, it was mostly in connection with full-time work, except among those who cared for someone in another household. Here, part-time work and seeking work were associated with providing care.

What do these findings mean? As before, we cannot be entirely sure that the patterns revealed are as a result of caring or whether they reflect, in some way, why people become carers.

As we have already pointed out, it is part of the received wisdom of the caring literature that being a carer has a substantial impact on paid employment, particularly if the carer is a woman. These findings confirm, certainly, that carers are less likely than non-carers to be in paid employment but there seems to be a more powerful effect (if effect it is) on male carers. However, the fact that male carers are more likely to be classed as seeking work, rather than as unable to work or keeping house, could suggest that men 'fill-in' as carers when unemployed. This may well be the case with different household carers where those seeking work are somewhat over-represented. However, there are other reasons to suggest that what we see here is a real effect on male carers' paid work.

First, evidence suggests that for a variety of reasons men are unlikely to take on alternative domestic or caring roles in the household when unemployed (Morris, 1987). Rather they maintain their perception of themselves as 'workers', even after substantial periods of unemployment. The ways in which men construct their lack of paid work and the benefit system considers them may thus explain why male carers in the GHS were more likely to be classed as 'seeking work'.

Secondly, other evidence suggests that younger male carers, particularly spouses, suffer threshold effects on their participation in paid work (Parker, 1989, 1993). Beyond a certain level of caring activity, they are unable to maintain full-time employment but, because of their relative lack of access to part-time work, withdraw from paid work entirely rather than, as women carers might do, take work with fewer hours. The extent to which this effect is evident, however, may be influenced both by the economic resources men are able to command from their employment (and thus their ability to pay for substitute care) and by their access to other caring inputs.

Patterns of paid work

So far we have looked at the different proportion of carers and non-carers who were in paid work or not. What differences, if any, were evident solely among those in paid work?

First, there was a significant difference in the incidence of full-time work between carers and non-carers. Carers were less likely overall than matched non-carers to be in full-time work (69 per cent and 74 per cent respectively) and more likely to be in part-time work (31 per cent and 26 per cent respectively). This pattern was evident among both female and male carers. Only two per cent of employed, male, non-carers were in part-time work compared to four per cent of male carers. Among employed females the comparable figures were 49 per cent and 56 per cent.

These patterns were much as might have been expected, given what was described earlier about carers' and non-carers' economic status. However, some crucial differences emerge when the analysis is taken further.

The only type of caring associated with differences in economic status between all working age carers and non-carers was the first type – *physical and personal care*. By contrast, among those in paid work it was only for those providing *physical not personal care* and *other practical help* that the significant differences in hours of work emerged.

Similarly, while among all carers it was only those providing help to someone in the same household who appeared to suffer effects on their labour market participation, among carers who were in paid work it was only those who looked after someone in a *different* household who showed significant differences in the hours worked.

Towards a model of the impact of caring on economic activity

What does this evidence suggest about the overall relationship between caring and economic activity?

Over and above the effects of age and sex (which are controlled for here) we know that providing care is related to reduced levels of participation in the labour market. However, it is providing the most intensive form of care, and caring for someone in the same household, that are most strongly influential. This tallies with much of what we know from earlier literature on caring. Unexpectedly, and contrary to what is found in the existing literature, women's overall level of labour market participation does not appear to be affected by caring to the same extent as is men's. Some reasons for the additional effects on men were rehearsed above. A possible reason for the relative lack of effect on women is that, in the now notorious phrase used in the 1974 White Paper, when talking about the reasons married women should not receive Invalid Care Allowance, 'they might be at home in any event' (House of Commons, 1974, §60, p. 20). Certainly, the proportions of female carers and non-carers overall who are classified as 'keeping house' vary little (30 per cent and 28 per cent respectively).

However, it is still the case that women providing the 'heaviest' forms of care are less likely than their peers to be in paid work and much more likely to be classed as 'keeping house'. For these two groups then, there is a real and measurable impact on labour market participation over and above that experienced by all women.

Further, the levels of paid employment for male and female carers in providing *personal and physical care* were very similar. It is the fact that *all* women are substantially less likely to be in paid employment usually because of their child-caring responsibilities, than *all* men, that makes the impact on male carers appear so much more substantial.

For those carers who do manage to maintain paid work the effects of caring are less clear cut. Although there is an overall tendency for carers to be working fewer hours than non-carers this does not vary by the type of care provided in the way that might have been expected. It is those providing 'middling' sorts of care who are least likely to be in full-time work, rather than those providing the heaviest types of care. There could be more than one reason for this.

First, it may be that people providing care of these less intensive types may have become carers because they were in part-time work, rather than have been in part-time work because of their caring responsibilities. Caring activities *physical not personal care* and *other practical help* take up less time than *personal and physical care* and *personal not physical care:* thus it may be feasible for these carers to maintain part-time work while also taking on caring responsibilities. By contrast, caring activities *practical help only* and *other help* take up so little time, on average, that maintaining full-time work at the same time as taking up caring is likely to present few problems.

A second and related possibility is that those most involved in caring, and who manage to stay in the labour market are in full-time work to the same degree as their peers *because* they are in full-time work. That is, the degree of care that has to be provided in the two most involved categories is so time-consuming that the only way to maintain contact with the labour market, for those who have main responsibility, is to earn enough to be able to afford to provide substitute care (Glendinning, 1992). This, for most people, means full-time work. Consequently, these working carers are involved in full-time employment to broadly the same extent as their peers.

Earnings and income

Personal earnings

Given carers' lower level of involvement in paid work it is not surprising to find that, overall, their personal earnings are lower than those of non-carers (Table 3.4). The average weekly personal earnings of all carers (£43) were significantly lower than those of all matched non-carers (£51). The size of the effect on personal earnings was, however, much greater for male than for female carers. On average, male carers had earnings some £16 per week lower than those of their non-carer peers. By contrast, female carers' earnings were, on average, £4 a week lower. However, the difference was statistically significant for both.

This effect on earnings was significant amongst those providing *personal and physical care, physical not personal care* and *other practical help*. The impact on those providing *personal and physical care* was because, as we saw above, they were less likely to be in any form of paid work. The impact on those providing *physical not personal care* and *other practical help* was explained by the greater likelihood of their being in part-time, rather than full-time, paid work.

Same-household carers' lower average earnings than matched non-carers (£31 compared to £46) also reflected the fact that they were less often in full-time paid work than their peers. The earnings of carers looking after someone in a different household, by contrast, were only slightly lower than those of matched non-carers (£47 compared with £53).

What of the earnings of those who *were* in paid work? Evidence from studies of those who look after their young disabled children has suggested that, all other things being equal, caring does affect the earnings of those who are able to remain in paid work (Baldwin, 1985; Pentol, 1983). Preliminary research with the carers of frail elderly people (Nissel and Bonnerjea, 1982) and an evaluation of the Invalid Care Allowance (McLaughlin, 1991) have suggested similar effects.

Table 3.4   Average personal earnings of all carers and matched non-carers: all carers with any personal earnings and matched non-carers by sex, type of care, and whether or not in same household

	Total matched sample		Total matched sample with any earnings	
	Carer £	Non-carer £	Carer £	Non-carer £
All	43	51 ***	86	96 ***
Male	71	87 ***	122	136 **
Female	24	28 **	55	62 **
Personal *and* physical care	27	42 **	77	91
Personal *not* physical care	38	43	86	86
Physical *not* personal care	35	53 **	75	98 *
Other practical help	48	54 *	90	99 *
Practical help only	40	48	80	95
Other help	50	53	90	100
In same household	31	46 ***	82	102 **
In different household	47	53 *	87	95 *

One-way analysis of variance (F) significant at 0.05 level (*), 0.01 level (**), or 0.001 level (***)

Clearly, even when carers were in paid work their average earnings were, overall, substantially lower than those of their non-carer peers (Table 3.4). This was the same regardless of whether the carers were male or female, or whether they provided care in the same household or elsewhere.

We saw earlier that when carers were in paid work, they were only marginally less likely than non-carers to be working full-time when providing personal care or when providing the least intensive forms of care. By contrast, those providing *physical not personal care* or *other practical help* were significantly less likely to be in full-time work than their peers. This pattern is reflected in the average earnings across the care types.

In sum, then, we can observe two different sorts of main effect on carers' personal earnings. First, among the most heavily involved, there is a depressive overall effect caused by the greater likelihood that they will not be in any form of paid work. Secondly, while those providing a 'middling' level of care are no more or less likely than their age/sex peers to have paid work, when they do work it is more likely to be part time. Consequently, their average earnings from paid work are lower. What we are not able to judge from the GHS data is whether or not carers in paid work also experienced a depressive effect on their *rates* of pay.

Personal income

Earnings from paid employment are not, of course, the only possible source of income for individuals. Social security benefit payments, income from savings or investments, rent payments from others in the household, occupational pensions and so on can all substitute for or supplement earnings from paid work. Few carers or non-carers (four per cent of each) had no form of personal income but the overall effect of carers' lower earnings was evident in the comparison between carers and non-carers.

Although very low, the average personal weekly income of female carers (£46) was little different from that of their peers (£49). For male carers, however, there was a substantial and significant difference of £12 a week (£98 carers, £110 non-carers). Same-household carers had significantly lower incomes than their non-carer equivalents (£58 and £73) but caring for someone in another household appeared to make little difference (£70 and £73 for carers and non-carers respectively). Within the different categories of caring the only significant differences found were among those providing *personal and physical care* and those providing *physical not personal care*. As we discuss below, this latter effect is explained by these carers having fewer hours of paid work but being unlikely to be compensated in any degree for this by the receipt of benefits.

Sources of personal income

The GHS records all sources of personal and household income and the amounts. This covers earnings from paid work, state social security provision, occupational benefits, maintenance, rent payments, savings income and any other short-term or long-term payments received from the state or elsewhere. There were relatively few differences between carers' and non-carers' sources of personal income (Table A5.1 in Appendix 5). Those that existed were, in some sense, expected.

As we have already seen, carers were less likely than non-carers to have income from earnings. By contrast, they were some-what more likely to be in receipt of invalidity benefit and attendance allowance. At first sight this latter finding seems strange. One might expect a higher proportion of *households* containing a carer to be in receipt of these two benefits but not carers them-selves. However, if we look further, some of the reasons for this become clear.

It is only among male carers and those carers who provide *practical help only* that invalidity benefit receipt is high. This could reflect the fact that male carers sometimes negotiate a 'sick role' for themselves in order to provide care (Parker, 1993) or that they are able to take on small amounts of caring activity if they leave the labour market for health reasons. Another possibility, that male carers are more likely to become ill because of or dur-ing caring, is not borne out by the data on ill-health and disabil-ity (see below).

The higher proportion of attendance allowance receipt found among carers was important only among the female carers and among those providing the heaviest types of care. This is likely to be explained by the fact that attendance allowance, although usually payable to the disabled person directly, is made payable to mothers when the disabled person is a minor or a suitable 'other' person if the recipient is suffering from dementia.

Male carers and those providing the heaviest forms of care were significantly more likely than their peers to be in receipt of sup-plementary benefit (SB), now income support, reflecting their generally lower participation in paid work. No differences between female carers and their peers were evident, by contrast. This probably reflects the fact that, all other things being equal, male carers without earnings from paid employment were more able to claim SB than were female carers. Many female carers are married; unless their husbands are also not in paid work they would be highly unlikely to have any right to SB. By contrast, most male carers who were not in paid employment, regardless of their marital status, would have a right to claim. Given that so many male carers, particularly those in the heaviest categories, were caring for wives who would not be earning, it was not surprising to find this over-representation of SB claimants.

The other major difference to emerge was in the role of savings. Same household carers and those providing the heaviest forms of care were substantially less likely than their non-carer equivalents to have income from savings. Given that age and sex are already controlled for this finding cannot reflect life-cycle or gender differences in capital accumulation. Rather, given its association with heavy forms of care and, therefore, with the longest caring 'histories', it is likely to reflect a real effect of being a carer. First, years of depressed earnings and income will inevitably have had an effect on carers' ability to save, as will any pressure to spend more because of the cared-for person's disability (Baldwin, 1985; Glendinning, 1992). Secondly, those who become carers in middle-age, particularly when this means giving up paid work, may find themselves propelled into an early 'old-age', using up savings which, had they not become carers, would not have been used until after retirement (Lewis and Meredith, 1988; Parker, 1993). Whichever effect is at play, it has clear and serious implications for carers' standard of living in their own old age.

Finally, it is worth pointing out that very few carers in the 1985 GHS received invalid care allowance (ICA). The survey was, of course, carried out before the extension of the ICA to married women but, even so, there is little evidence of its reaching other groups. This is not so surprising when overlapping benefit regulations mean that those without paid work who claim social security benefits are unlikely to gain financially from receipt of ICA (see McLaughlin, 1991 for a full exploration of this effect).

Household income
So far we have looked only at the carers' own income. For those carers who lived with other people – whether the cared-for person or others – the concept of household income is also useful for making comparisons with non-carers.

Household income is not, of course, an unproblematic concept. We know that not all members of a household necessarily have equal access to all the income that household commands (Pahl,

1989; Wilson, 1987). Further, we are starting to understand that, within households containing a carer and a cared-for person, conventional notions of financial dependence and independence may be inadequate. In some cases disabled people who are, notionally at least, financially 'dependent' may be supporting their carer and vice versa (Glendinning, 1992; McLaughlin, 1991). However, looking at household income does give us an opportunity to see whether other household members' contributions *could* balance the deficits caused by carers' depressed earnings and incomes, if all members actually had equal access to and use of that household income.

One interpretative difficulty in examining household income is that carers and non-carers, as explained earlier, live in significantly different-sized households. We have controlled for this difference in two ways here; by presenting straight per capita household income[6] and by using an equivalent income scale, the Luxembourg Income Scale.[7]

The per capita income comparison shows that, overall, carers' household income was significantly lower than that of equivalent non-carers. However, when different sub-groups are compared it becomes clear that it was only among male carers, those providing *personal and physical care*, those providing *physical not personal care* and same-household carers that the differences remain significant (Table 3.5).

When equivalent incomes (which control both for household size and household composition) are used, even fewer differences between carers' and non-carers' household incomes are evident (Table 3.6).

Regardless of household size or composition, then, we can see that carers' households have lower incomes than non-carers' households. While there is no longer any significant difference between households with male or female carers, it is still the case that particular types of caring activity, and caring for someone in the same household, are associated with lower incomes.

---

6 Per capita household income is calculated by dividing total household income by the number of people, including dependent children, in the household.

7 The Luxembourg Income Scale uses the following values to calculate equivalent incomes:

A single adult	1.00
A couple	1.50
A couple and one child	2.00
A couple and two children	2.50
A couple and three children	3.00
Single parent and one child	1.50
Single parent and two children	2.00

Table 3.5   Per capita income of carers and matched non-carers: overall, by sex, by type of care, and by whether or not in same household

	Carer £	Non-carer £
Overall	61	64 **
Male	62	67 *
Female	59	62
Personal *and* physical care	53	67 ***
Personal *not* physical care	59	61
Physical *not* personal care	54	66 **
Other practical help	63	64
Practical help only	62	60
Other help	67	64
In same household	50	64 ***
In different household	64	64

One way analysis of variance (F) sig at 0.05 level (*), 0.01 level (**) or 0.001 level (***)

Table 3.6   Equivalent incomes (LIS) of carers and matched non-carers: overall, by sex, by type of care, and by whether or not in same household

	Carer £	Non-carer £
Overall	84	88 *
Male	86	92
Female	82	86
Personal *and* physical care	75	90 **
Personal *not* physical care	84	83
Physical *not* personal care	75	90 **
Other practical care	86	89
Practical help only	83	82
Other help	92	88
In same household	72	86 ***
In different household	88	89

One-way analysis of variance (F) sig at 0.05 level (*) .01 level (**) or 0.001 level (***)

It is possible that these findings reflect two different sorts of effect. First, the lower equivalent incomes of carers in the first caring category are most likely due to the lower likelihood of these carers having any sort of paid work, and the inability of the benefits they or other household members receive (in greater proportions than their non-carer equivalents – see Table A5.2, Appendix 5) to compensate fully for this. By contrast, those in the third caring category, particularly men, are no less likely to be in paid work but, when they are, are significantly more likely to work part-time. Their personal receipt of benefits, however, is no more than their non-carer equivalents. Further, their households, as a whole, are no more likely than equivalent non-carer households to receive major income-replacement benefits such as the state pension and supplementary benefit or disability-related benefits such as attendance allowance. Carers in this category thus fall between two stools. They have not (yet) given up full-time work, and therefore they fail to qualify for income replacement benefits. On the other hand, other members of their household, for whom they may be caring, appear to be insufficiently disabled to qualify for compensatory benefits related to disability.

Assets

If certain types of carers have lower incomes than their non-carer equivalents, one might expect them to have fewer domestic assets and consumer durables in their households. Alternatively, because of the particular demands of caring, they might have *more* of some assets, such as washing machines.

On an initial comparison between carers and matched non-carers there were few differences in household possession of assets. Only in relation to washing machines and cars was there any difference and, in both cases, carers were significantly more likely to own these than were non-carers. Possession of all other goods covered by the GHS – central heating, TV, video, refrigerator, freezer, clothes dryer, dishwasher, telephone and computer – was more or less identical for the two groups. Both male and female carers were more likely than their peers to have a washing machine but only females were more likely to have access to a car.

So far, this is as one might expect; both washing machines and cars are items that one might expect disabled people and their families to have more need of. However, when the data are broken down into care types and same or different household carers we find that it is not the most heavily involved carers who have these extra assets. Only carers providing *other practical help* and *other help* were in households that were more likely to have a car. Only where carers were providing *other practical help* were carer households more likely than non-carer households to possess a washing machine. Further, it was different household carers, not same-household carers, who had more of these assets than their non-carer peers.

Given the nature of the care being provided in the first three categories – the heavy personal and physical tending associated with high degrees of impairment – it is disturbing to find that these carers did not have greater access than their peers to two assets that would undoubtedly have made their lives easier. Knowing what we do about their income levels, however, the finding is less surprising.

There is one *caveat* to be made about the interpretation of these findings. Although the level of possession of domestic assets and durables differs little between carers and matched non-carers, we know nothing about the quality or appropriateness of the equipment. For example, we do not know whether heavily involved carers are more likely to have, say, automatic washing machines when their peers may have less expensive twin-tubs. We do not know whether carers have to spend more on maintaining their cars or have to replace them more often to ensure reliability. Conversely, we do not know whether or not carers are able to replace worn out or old-fashioned equipment at the same rate as their peers. The smaller-scale literature on the impact of caring tells us that both these sorts of processes occur (see, for example, Baldwin, 1985 and Glendinning, 1992) but, in the cross-sectional approach offered by the GHS, we cannot identify them directly.

Housing and tenure

In a society where increasing importance is placed on owner-occupation as a stepping stone to major capital accumulation, the level of home ownership is, clearly, a useful 'outcome measure' on which to compare carers and non-carers.

Overall, there was no difference in the type of accommodation carers lived in, compared with matched non-carers. Nor was there any significant difference in the proportions who were living in owner-occupied premises (63 per cent carers, 66 per cent non-carers). Male carers were just as likely as their non-carer equivalents, and female carers as likely as their equivalents, to be in owner-occupied homes.

However, significant differences were evident in certain categories of caring and among same-household carers. Carers in the first two categories were less likely than their counterparts to be in owner-occupied housing (54 per cent and 67 per cent, and 56 and 66 per cent respectively). Similarly, same household carers were significantly less likely than non-carers to be in owner-occupied homes (55 per cent and 63 per cent respectively).

Some of this difference probably reflects the differences, seen above, in income and employment status of heavily involved carers compared to non-carers. Both prolonged low income and status as a benefit recipient are likely to depress the likelihood of becoming an owner-occupier. Further, sharing a household with a disabled person who, him- or herself, may be unlikely to be in paid work, must depress this likelihood further.

Overall, carers were more likely to be living in overcrowded housing, as measured by the bedroom standard.[8] The vast majority of households in Great Britain (96 per cent) are now equal to or well above the bedroom standard (Foster *et al.*, 1990). Carers, by contrast, are more likely to be living in households which are crowded than are their non-carer peers (seven per cent and four per cent respectively). This difference does not apply to all sorts of carers. Women carers, carers providing *personal and physical care*, and those who lived in the same household as the person being cared for were the only sub-groups of carers who were significantly more likely than their non-carer equivalents to be in overcrowded households. Seven per cent of female carers lived in households below the bedroom standard, compared with only three per cent of their peers. Similarly, nine per cent of carers providing *personal and physical care* and 13 per cent of same-household carers were in below standard households compared to three per cent, in both cases, of their non-carer equivalents.

These findings are, perhaps, not so surprising given the significantly greater household size found among carers generally (see above). However, it was not solely larger household size that

---

[8] The bedroom standard 'is used to estimate occupation density by allocating a standard number of bedrooms to each household in accordance with its age/sex/marital status composition and the relationship of the members to one another' (1985 GHS, Appendix A, p. 126). This measure is then used to express the difference in the actual number of bedrooms in the household from the 'standard'.

accounted for overcrowding. Those providing *personal not physical care* and *other help*, and different-household carers, were also in large households, but not overcrowded.

A number of possibilities suggest themselves, the most likely of which is that carers in certain sub-groups are not able to respond to the greater pressure of numbers in their households because of their more limited financial situation and/or because they are renting their accommodation. If owner-occupiers they cannot 'trade-up'; if in rented accommodation they may be unable to negotiate more spacious housing or be unable to contemplate owner-occupation which might give them more space.[9]

Health and disability

The relationship between physical health and caring is one of the most problematic in the literature on informal care. On the one hand, small-scale projects repeatedly reveal that carers feel that their health has been adversely affected by caring. On the other hand there has been no sufficiently large or well-enough designed research which could conclusively underline the link between physical ill-health and the burdens of caring (Parker, 1990a).

There are a number of reasons for this. First, women are generally less physically well than men, often due to the aftermath of child-birth. This effect is shown year after year in the GHS. If a higher proportion of 'heavy end' carers are women (and we have seen from the earlier chapters that this is so) then, clearly, caring and physical ill-health will be linked, although not necessarily causally.

Secondly, older people are generally less well physically than younger people; another effect revealed annually in the GHS. People over the age of 45 are more likely than younger people to

---

[9] Another possible explanation is to do with household composition. Same-sex adolescents (10–20 years of age) and children under ten are 'paired' in assessing the bedroom standard; that is they are 'allocated' a shared bedroom. By contrast, those over the age of 20, other than married couples, are 'allocated' a bedroom each. Even when they have the same number of bedrooms, households containing high proportions of children to adults are less likely as a whole to have bedroom standards below the standard than are households containing high proportions of adults to children. *All* types of carers were more likely to be in households with more adults. However, this effect seemed more pronounced among female carers, those providing *personal and physical care* and in-household carers. This is probably insufficient of itself to account for all the overcrowding effect, but clearly contributes to it.

be carers. Hence, again, caring and physical ill-health are linked but one does not necessarily cause the other.

Thirdly, we do know that emotional stress and caring responsibilities are linked, although the key characteristics of the carer's or cared-for person's situation which *cause* stress have not been unequivocally demonstrated (Parker, 1990a). High levels of emotional stress may make the symptoms of physical ill-health more prominent to the sufferer or more difficult to cope with. In such situations, carers may interpret physical ill-health which would have occurred anyway as due to, or exacerbated by, caring responsibilities.

The 1985 GHS offers the first opportunity to examine these issues in a controlled way although the cause and effect issue cannot be wholly resolved because of the cross-sectional nature of the data. All GHS respondents were asked about their general health over the previous 12 months. As Table 3.7 shows, although carers were less likely than matched non-carers to say that their health was good, the difference was not substantial, given the size of the two groups.

Table 3.7   General health of carers and matched non-carers

General health	Carer %	Non-carer %	All %
Good	59	62	60
Fairly good	29	26	27
Not good	13	12	12
Base (100%)	2,514	2,514	5,028

$X^2 = 7.8$, df = 2, $p < 0.05$

Within sub-groups, there were no differences between carers and non-carers related to sex, category of care or different-household care. Only between same-household carers and their equivalents was any significant difference in health status recorded (Table 3.8).

The relationship with place of caring is, perhaps, mediated by the experience of emotional stress. Although the GHS collects no information on stress it seems intuitively likely that, all other things being equal, providing care in the same household might be more stressful than providing it elsewhere. This seems especially likely given the over-crowding in such house-

holds revealed earlier. The importance of spatial arrangements
within households, in order to allow carers to maintain bound-
aries round their lives, is only just being recognised (Twigg and
Atkin, 1993).

Table 3.8   General health of same-household carers and
matched non-carers

| General health | Same household | | |
	Carer %	Non-carer %	All %
Good	51	60	55
Fairly good	31	27	29
Not good	18	14	16
Base (100%)	726	726	1,452

$X^2 = 11.4$, df = 2, p < 0.01

We also know that same household carers are less likely than
their non-carer equivalents to be in paid work, another factor
which may affect their emotional state and, thereby, their perception of their physical health. Another possibility is that we
are observing a 'survivor' effect amongst heavily involved carers; that is, heavily involved carers with substantial health
problems of their own may have ceased their caring activity
altogether or reduced it to a lower level. This would have the
effect of lowering the level of reported ill-health among those
in the 'heavy end' categories.

The GHS, in addition to the question on general health in the
previous 12 months, has a question about any *long-standing* illness, disability or infirmity. Here, there were some clear differences between carers and non-carers but not those that might
have been expected. Some 40 per cent of carers said that they
suffered from some long-standing illness or disability, compared
to 36 per cent of non-carers. Although relatively small, this difference was statistically significant. However, the difference was
evident only among women. Male carers and their non-carer
peers were similarly likely to report a long-standing condition
while female carers were more likely than female non-carers to
do so.

One might have expected, as with general health, that the most
heavily involved carers would be most likely to report problems. But, again, this was not so. It was those providing *physical*

not personal care, other practical help and *other help* who were more likely than their non-carer equivalents to report chronic ill-health or disability. Because carers in these categories were more likely to be helping someone in a different household, there was also a difference with different household but not same household carers.

On the face of it, these findings are puzzling. First, we know that neither age nor sex differences between carers and non-carers in each of the sub-groups can account for them. Secondly, as with recent general health, if a caring effect *was* present one might expect it to be present most obviously among the most heavily involved carers. This, as we have seen, was not the case.

One possibility is that these findings, rather than reflecting the effect of caring on carers, actually help to explain *why* certain people become carers. To understand this we need to go back to the information on economic status.

Despite being more likely than non-carers to report some disability or long-standing illness, carers providing *physical not personal care, other practical help* and *other help* were no more likely to report that they were unable to work. This suggests, perhaps, that their illness or disability was not severely limiting. However, when they were in paid work, carers in the first two of these three categories were significantly less likely than non-carers to be working full-time. Perhaps, then, people in these categories have time available to provide help at a low level, because they are at home as a result of an illness or disability that is not seriously limiting. It must be stressed that this is a very tentative suggestion, based on differences between carers and non-carers that are statistically significant but not strikingly so. However, it is an issue which may deserve future exploration in empirical research.

Conclusion

The GHS data offer an unprecedented opportunity to test some of the 'effects' of informal caring previously identified in small-scale research. Although the cross-sectional nature of the survey limits to some degree the interpretation and extrapolation that are possible from the analysis, the age/sex matching process allows reasonable confidence to be placed on the findings.

The most significant steps forward in our understanding of the impact of caring lie in the areas of finance and health. First, the analysis has shown that carers as a whole, and particularly those providing the most intense forms of care and caring for someone in the same household, suffer effects on their labour market participation and, thereby, on their personal earnings and income. Even when in paid work, carers earn less than their non-carer peers, regardless of whether they are male or female, or whether they provide care in the same household or elsewhere. These effects carry through into household income, indicating that other household members' incomes (if any) are not able to make up the 'deficit' caused by carers' depressed earnings and incomes. Carers are far less likely than their peers to have income from savings, indicating that depressed incomes may have a life-long effect.

The income effect of caring appears to carry over into housing tenure and conditions for some groups of carers, meaning that they have less access to owner-occupation and are more likely to be in overcrowded conditions.

The second step forward in our understanding is in relation to carers' physical health. The analysis has suggested that previous research which has argued a causal relationship between caring and current physical ill-health may have confounded the effects of caring with those of age and sex, both of which also influence health status. Female carers were slightly more likely than their peers to report a long-standing illness or disability, but this was among the least heavily involved carers. This suggests that some people may take on low-level caring or helping responsibilities because they are at home more due to an illness or disability that is not particularly limiting. This is clearly an area which deserves further investigation in research specifically designed to examine it.

Carers and services

Introduction

Despite growing awareness of the role of informal carers in helping disabled or frail people to live in the community (see Chapter One), there are relatively few services within existing structures which have the explicit aim of supporting carers themselves. On the one hand, conventional service provision is typically seen as being 'for' the disabled or frail person; support which accrues to the carer is thus often a secondary, and sometimes unintentional, result. On the other hand, the few developments which have had carers as their specific target are usually too small and localized to make any impression on the majority of carers (Twigg *et al.*, 1990; Twigg, 1989; Parker, 1990a).

Previous research has suggested that conventional services – home help, meals-on-wheels, bathing services – go predominantly to those disabled or frail people who live alone. When services *do* go to households which contain an informal carer they are often crisis-orientated rather than part of long-term support. Further, the criteria by which services are allocated are often irrational (not allocated in relation to need) and discriminatory (not provided where female carers, particularly married women, are available) (Parker, 1990a).

No large-scale research evidence exists about the views of carers: either about the services that they and those they care for receive; or about those they would like to receive. However, a series of small-scale, often qualitative, studies are starting to give a clearer idea of what range of support services carers would find helpful (Parker, 1990a; Twigg, 1992; Twigg and Atkin, 1993). Coupled with a number of 'carers' initiatives' these identify a 'core' of services and advice for informal carers:

- information and advice about caring
- assessment and review of carers' needs and those of the person they care for
- financial support

- training
- help in the tasks of caring, including respite care
- emotional support

(King's Fund Informal Caring Programme, 1988)

Although it is useful to identify core services in this way, it is also clear from research that any *individual* carer's needs will be determined by her or his personal circumstances – age, sex, household composition, labour market participation and so on. For example, the form that adequate practical help might take for an elderly man caring for a frail wife is likely to be different from that for a younger single women, in paid work, caring for a frail mother. Similarly, the support required by a young married couple where one partner has a physical disability and where both are in paid work is likely to be different, both in form and quantity, from that required by a lone parent caring for a multiply disabled, pre-school child.

Further, certain types of support may interact with, and influence the need for, other types. For example, a young woman caring for a pre-school disabled child may prefer to receive a package of substitute care for her child, to enable her to take paid work, rather than receive an income replacement benefit. Or an elderly man caring for a frail wife may prefer to receive direct domiciliary services rather than be given money to enable him to arrange and pay for such services himself. Currently, of course, such choices are not widely available to carers, if at all (Twigg and Atkin, 1993).

Service receipt and the General Household Survey

One of the questions asked of those who identified themselves as providing care or help in the 1985 GHS was whether or not the person they assisted also received help from a range of statutory and voluntary health and social services.

This question revealed substantial differences in service receipt between carers who lived in the same household as the person being cared for and those who lived elsewhere. People whose carer lived elsewhere were twice as likely to receive regular visits from their GP or a social worker, four times as likely to have a home help, and ten times as likely to receive meals-on-wheels as were those whose carers were in the same household[10] (Green, 1988).

---

[10] Where the person being cared for was the 'main dependant', as defined in the 1985 GHS.

This original analysis leaves a number of issues to be explored, however. First, the 'living alone' effect has to be teased out. A high proportion of those whose carer was in a different household lived alone. We already know that some services go preferentially to those who live alone. It may be, therefore, that the observed difference in service receipt is due to this effect rather than to whether or not the *carer* is in the same household.

Secondly, there is the issue of service substitutability. A series of large-scale surveys of disability and old age, from Harris (1971) onwards, has shown that living with others affects not only whether any services are received at all but also appears to influence the provision of particular services. Briefly, this evidence suggests some form of 'hierarchy' of service provision, by which carers in the same household are apparently less likely to be expected to attend to the nursing care of disabled and older people than to cook their meals or do their housework (Parker, 1990a).

Arber's analysis of the 1980 GHS (which like the 1985 survey, had a section for older people) has developed the notion of 'substitutability', that is, the extent to which informal carers can and do substitute for formal services (Arber *et al.*, 1988). This showed that domestic services for elderly people are 'substitutable' by any available carer, while personal health and hygiene services are only partially substitutable, depending upon the relationship between the carer and the cared-for person. Elderly married couples in the 1980 GHS appeared to perform for one another 'at least some of the functions otherwise carried out by a district nurse' (Arber *et al.*, 1988, p. 169). By contrast, a relationship between generations *and* across the sexes, made a substantial difference. District nursing support was twice as likely to be provided 'where the unmarried adult carer [was] caring for an elderly person of the opposite sex' (p. 169) as where it was a person of the same sex being cared for.

Thirdly, there is the related issue of sex of the carer. Early research in this field suggested that women carers were, across the board, less likely to receive services (or, more accurately, the person they were looking after was less likely to receive services) than were male carers. More recently, Arber and her colleagues (Arber *et al.*, 1988; Arber and Gilbert, 1989) have demonstrated that it is not sex, *per se*, which influences service provision but rather the inter-relationships between sex of the carer, sex of the cared-for person, household composition and size, the relationship between the carer and cared-for person,

the carer's relationship to the labour market, and the substitutability of the service itself. In addition, Arber's analysis was
able to take into account the extent of the cared-for person's
need for support.

When this had been controlled for, younger, lone, female carers
of elderly people were found to be no less likely than their male
equivalents to receive support. However, *married* women carers
under 65 years of age received the lowest levels of domestic and
personal health care support. Further, elderly men and women
who lived alone were over five times more likely to receive a
home help service than were elderly married couples, regardless of who was the carer. Whether or not similar patterns
emerge when carers of all types and ages are included is
explored in this chapter, as is the 'living alone' effect, and substitutability.

Defining a need for services

There is a substantial difficulty with interpretation of the GHS
data in relation to service provision. This arises because no
information was collected from informal carers about the
degree of impairment of those they assisted or the extent of
their need for help. Rather, carers were asked what help they
provided. This may be a weak guide to the need for services for
three reasons.

First, where the carer was not the *sole* person involved in helping a particular individual, the range of helping tasks actually
involved in supporting that individual might be substantially
different from that supplied by the carer identified in the GHS.
For example, a GHS carer might have reported keeping an eye
on the helped person and taking him or her out. Yet it is possible that some other carer might have been providing intense
personal or physical care to the same person. Only in a limited
number of circumstances is it possible to use the GHS data to
link people caring for the same person in order to get a more
complete picture of the whole range of help he or she received.

Secondly, there is some evidence that, among elderly people at
least, help 'needed' may reflect the *availability* of help rather than
degree of disability and that the availability of help is, in turn,
affected by household composition (Wenger, 1986). We also
know that the 'need' for help with certain domestic tasks can be
determined socially: elderly women struggle longer to maintain
household responsibilities when living with unmarried sons
than when with unmarried daughters (Wright, 1983); men are

more likely to 'need' help with domestic tasks than are women; and women are more likely to 'need' help with household maintenance tasks (Wenger, 1986; Qureshi, 1986; Parker, 1993). Even if we knew the full range of tasks provided to individuals, then, this would still be a less than perfect guide to their level of impairment and their 'need' for support.

Thirdly, service receipt itself may determine or alter the carer's level of involvement and the tasks undertaken. For example, receipt of home help and bathing services may mean that the informal carer of a substantially disabled person may become involved only in relatively 'light' caring. Absence of those services may mean that he or she becomes heavily involved.

These interpretive problems may be responsible for some of the somewhat paradoxical findings about service receipt reported in the 1985 GHS report (Green, 1988). Here, as we have already mentioned, cared-for people living in a different household from the carer were reported to be more likely to have received services even though, as a group, they were less likely to be receiving the more intense forms of care from the carers.

One way round this difficulty is to change the nature of the question asked of the data. Instead of asking whether services appear to discriminate against people with comparable levels of need when they have an informal carer, we can ask whether services appear to discriminate between carers providing similar types and levels of care and, if so, on what basis. This approach does not, of course, solve the problem of those informal carers who provide 'more' care than the person being helped 'really needs'. It does, however, allow us to ask strategic questions about the role of services in supporting carers in the tasks they actually carry out.

In the remainder of this chapter, we look first at all the carers identified in the 1985 GHS and the pattern of service provision to those whom they were helping. In the following chapter, however, we will attempt to address the more strategic question of support for informal carers by restricting the analysis to the most heavily involved carers as defined by typology of caring developed in the first chapter.

Service receipt in the whole group

The 1985 GHS contains information about 'regular visits at least once a month' to the person helped by informal carers, from a range of professionals or services.

These are:

- doctor
- community or district nurse
- health visitor
- social worker
- home help
- meals-on-wheels
- voluntary workers
- other professional visitor or service

In addition, chiropodists and wardens were mentioned sufficiently often under the 'other' category to be given separate codes in the original analysis.

Fewer than half of the people being cared for were receiving any service at all. Among those who were, visits from a home help or doctor were the most common, followed by a community or district nurse (Table 4.1). Very few people were receiving more than one service (Table 4.2).

Table 4.1   Range of services received by cared-for people

Type of service	% receiving service
Home help	24
Doctor	22
Nurse	15
Meals-on-wheels	8
Health visitor	6
Social worker	6
Voluntary worker	4
Warden (sheltered accommodation)	2
Chiropodist	1
Other	5
Base	3,032

Table 4.2: Number of services received by cared-for people

Number of services	% receiving
0	54
1	21
2	14
3	6
4	3
5	1
6	<1
7	<1
Base	3,032

In order to simplify this stage of the analysis, we grouped the ten services into five categories, according to the *type* of service provided. These are:

i.   Medical care (doctor)
ii. Personal care (nurse/chiropodist)
iii. Advice (health visitor/social worker)
iv. Domestic help (home help/meals-on-wheels)
v.   Other (voluntary worker/warden/other).

Obviously these categories are not entirely distinct. District nurses may provide some services that are more properly thought of as medical; some home help services now provide forms of personal care; social workers may arrange services as well as provide support and advice; and voluntary workers may provide a whole range of different sorts of help. Further, respondents may have confused the source of different sorts of help. For example, there is a lot of confusion among elderly people, particularly, about the respective roles of community nurses and health visitors. However, we felt that there was sufficient separation, in practice, between the care services provided to warrant the groupings.

In the following sub-sections we look at the distribution of these five types of service by the carer's sex, age, marital status, whether or not the carer and cared-for person were the same sex, employment status, health, relationship to the cared-for person, level of responsibility, and by the type of care provided and whether it was provided in the same or a different household.

Here and throughout this chapter the X^2 statistic was used to test whether the distributions observed varied significantly from those expected. Where statistically significant differences were observed this is indicated by the use of asterisks: one for a result significant at the 0.5 level, two at the 0.01 level, and three for the 0.001 level or beyond. NS indicates that no statistically significant difference was observed.

Sex, age and marital status of carer

Table 4.3 compares the receipt of different services by cared-for people by whether their carer was male or female. Medical services were the only ones to show any significant difference. Those being cared for by women were slightly more likely to be seeing a doctor regularly. Given that women were somewhat more likely than men to be caring for very elderly people, and that very elderly people have more contact with their GPs than young ones (Foster *et al.*, 1990) this may explain the difference.

Table 4.3   Receipt of services by sex of carer

| | Sex of carer | | |
| | M | F | |
Type of service	% receiving service		
Medical	20	23	*
Personal	16	16	NS
Domestic	27	26	NS
Advice	10	10	NS
Other	9	10	NS
Any service	46	48	NS
Minimum base	1,133	1,727	

By contrast, receipt of all services except 'other' was significantly related to age of the carer (Table 4.4). Carers in the older age groups were more likely to be looking after people receiving any service, particularly personal and domestic services. Again this relationship may be explained by the ages of the cared-for people. Carers aged 65 or over were somewhat over-represented among those caring for individuals who were also over 65, and significantly over-represented among those caring for people aged 76 and over.

Carers who were widowed were more likely than other carers to be looking after someone who received any service, who saw a

Table 4.4   Receipt of services by age of carer

Type of service	Age group of carer							
	16–25	26–35	36–45	46–55	56–65	66–75	76+	
	% receiving service							
Medical	26	23	18	21	21	26	30	*
Personal	19	13	17	14	15	23	18	**
Domestic	28	22	22	26	26	33	36	***
Advice	10	13	8	8	9	12	17	*
Other	10	11	11	10	8	10	10	NS
Any service	51	45	45	45	47	55	54	*
Minimum base	218	361	633	669	553	317	102	

doctor regularly or who received some form of domestic help. This, again, seems likely to reflect an age effect; the likelihood of being widowed increasing with age.

Sex of carer and sex of cared-for person

There was substantial variation in service receipt depending on the sex of the carer in relation to sex of the cared-for person. Where women were caring for men service receipt was at its lowest in relation to all services except 'other'. By contrast, service receipt was highest in relation to all except advice services when a woman was caring for another woman (Table 4.5).

Table 4.5   Receipt of services by sex of carer/sex of cared-for person

| Type of service | Sex of carer/sex of cared-for person | | | |
| | Female/ female | Male/ male | Male/ female | Female/ male |
	% receiving service			
Medical	26	20	20	18 ***
Personal	18	16	17	13 *
Domestic	29	26	27	19 ***
Advice	11	13	9	7 *
Other	12	7	10	7 *
Any service	52	49	46	40 ***
Minimum base	1,127	300	826	594

In all cases where women were looking after men, service receipt was at a lower level than where men were looking after women.

The biggest difference between these groups of 'cross-sex' carers was in relation to domestic services where 27 per cent of male carers were looking after a woman who received some form of domestic service, compared to 19 per cent of women carers who were looking after a man who received some form of domestic service.

Employment status

Receipt of domestic, advice and 'other' services varied with the employment status of the carer. Retired carers were more likely to be helping someone who received domestic help, reflecting yet again the age effect of those being cared for. Receipt of advice services was more common when carers were keeping house, and receipt of 'other' services when the carer had paid employ-

Table 4.6 Receipt of services by relationship between carer and cared-for person

Type of service	Relationship of cared-for person to carer					
	Neighbour	'Other' relative	Parent-in-law	Parent	Spouse	Child
			% receiving service			
Medical	33	25	19	20	14	6 ***
Personal	21	20	16	14	11	9 ***
Domestic	46	27	28	21	11	4 ***
Advice	16	9	8	8	6	14 ***
Other	13	12	10	8	7	8 *
Any service	66	52	46	42	31	26 ***
Minimum base	544	518	386	956	285	166

ment. Overall, however, those whose carers were in paid work or classed as 'other' economically inactive,[11] were less likely than others to be receiving *any* service.

Health of the carer

Advice services were the only ones where receipt varied with the health of the carer. Those who said that their health was not good were significantly more likely to be caring for someone who received visits from a health visitor or social worker. There is a possibility, again, that age of the carer is playing an intervening role here.

Relationship between the carer and the cared-for person

One of the major variables which previous research has found to influence service receipt among carers is the nature of the relationship between the carer and the cared-for person (see above). Taken in isolation from any other variables, Table 4.6 shows that people were far more likely to receive all the services covered when they were being looked after by a non-relative.

Further, in those situations where a spouse or child was being cared for, receipt of medical, personal and domestic services was at a particularly low level.

These patterns are likely to reflect a number of factors, either individually or in combination. First, those helping friends or neighbours were, obviously, most likely to be doing this in a household other than their own. As was mentioned earlier, the original GHS report showed that service receipt was much more common among those whose carer lived in a different household (Green, 1988, Table 5.8). Secondly, people with carers in a different household were, overall, substantially older than those whose carer was in the same household (Green, 1988, Figure 3C) and thus more likely to receive some services. Thirdly, when people have carers who live elsewhere they are, by definition, more likely to live alone than those whose carer is in the same household. We already know that, overall, services may go more often to people who live alone.

---

[11] Other than retired, keeping house or a student.

More importantly, perhaps, Table 4.6 shows us which people are very *unlikely* to get services. Those being cared for by a spouse, parent, or child were much less likely than others to receive services despite the fact that these groups were most likely to involve carers in the most intense forms of care (see Chapter Two).

Level of responsibility for the cared-for person

As would be expected, given what has gone before, service receipt varied significantly with the level of responsibility carried by the carer (Table 4.7).

Table 4.7   Receipt of services by level of responsibility of carers

	Level of responsibility				
Type of service	Sole carer	Main carer	Joint main carer	Not main carer	
	% receiving service				
Medical	17	20	15	30	***
Personal	12	15	10	23	***
Domestic	21	24	21	32	***
Advice	8	9	6	13	***
Other	7	8	9	14	***
Any service	38	43	37	59	***
Minimum base	632	823	308	989	

In all types of service, those people whose carers did not carry the main responsibility for them were more likely to be in receipt than were others. People who had only one carer or whose carer shared responsibility were particularly unlikely to be receiving domestic, medical or personal services.

At first sight these findings seem worrying but they do require careful interpretation. First, those without main responsibility for the person being helped were less likely to live in the same household. As we have seen above, for a number of reasons this is likely to affect service provision. Secondly, if those carers did not have main responsibility others must have been involved in providing care. In some cases this may have been a paid helper but in others would have been an informal carer.

Table 4.8   Receipt of services by type of care provided

Type of service	Category of care					
	1	2	3	4	5	6	
				% receiving service			
Medical	25	19	33	21	18	23	***
Personal	26	21	23	13	12	17	***
Domestic	22	21	24	29	18	27	***
Advice	9	12	13	9	7	12	NS
Other	10	13	10	10	4	11	NS
Any service	51	47	54	46	36	49	**
Minimum base	363	270	228	1,412	205	371	

This carer would thus be looking after someone who was receiving a service.

The typology developed in Chapter Two distinguished well between different sorts of carers and between different levels of involvement in caring. Therefore, one might expect it also to be related to different patterns of service receipt. As Table 4.8 shows, this was the case.

These data suggest a rather more targeted delivery of services than has been obvious so far. For example, those people whose informal carers provided both *personal and physical care* were more likely than others to be receiving formal personal care services. Those whose informal carers provided them with *other practical help* were more likely than others to be getting formal domestic services. Among those receiving *physical not personal care*, however, the relatively high level of personal care services may suggest substitution effects: that is, personal care is provided from formal rather than informal sources.

The higher level of receipt of medical services among people receiving *physical not personal care* may reflect the fact that as we saw in Chapter Two, the main impairments in this group were physical. While being physically disabled does not mean that an individual is ill, it may well be associated with a higher level of need for medical surveillance to prevent complications such as skin sores, kidney infections and so on.

In sum, two different sorts of effect seem to be evident from these data. First, we can see that some forms of service apparently supplement the type of care in which informal carers are already involved. The second effect appears to be a real substitution effect where services input means that the carer does not become involved in particular types of care. These apparent effects, and their relationship to other characteristics of the carer and the person being helped, will be explored in more detail below.

This analysis also suggests that type of care provided may be a rather better proxy for the level of 'need' for care than the discussion in the introduction suggested it might be.

Living in the same household
We have already seen that whether care is provided in the carer's own household or elsewhere is significantly related to service receipt. This is the same for all forms of service. However, it is worth looking again at the patterns of receipt

because some services are more strongly associated with where care is provided than are others (Table 4.9).

Receipt of a personal care service, although still significantly more likely when the carer is looking after someone in another household, is much less strongly related to where care is provided than other services. By contrast, the largest difference in the receipt of services is found with domestic services. The implications of these differences, which suggest some form of hierarchy of substitutability as discussed in the introduction, are explored in more detail in the next chapter.

Table 4.9   Receipt of services by whether or not cared-for person lives in the same household as the carer

	Cared-for person lives in:		
	Same household	Different household	
Type of service	% receiving service		
Medical	12	26	***
Personal	14	17	*
Domestic	7	33	***
Advice	7	11	***
Other	5	11	***
Any service	29	54	***
Minimum base	754	2,109	

Conclusion

The analysis presented in this chapter has shown that there are some substantial variations in service receipt among cared-for people. Some of these differences, for example those related to the age of the carer or the type of care provided, are as might be expected. Others, for example those related to the carers' marital status or relationship to the cared-for person, are not. Conversely, there were some areas where a *lack* of variation in service receipt was more surprising. Given all that has been written about male and female carers, one might have expected substantial differences in service receipt between them but this was not immediately evident. One might also have expected those carers who were in poor health to receive domestic or personal services more often than others but, again, this was not so.

However, as indicated from time to time through the chapter, the patterns revealed may be strongly influenced by intervening variables. In the next chapter we attempt to tease out some of these effects by applying multi-variate statistical techniques.

Accounting for variations in service receipt

Introduction

One of the difficulties with the straightforward, variable-by-variable, account of service receipt given in Chapter Four is the substantial inter-relationships between a number of those variables. For example, *where* care is received is closely related to the relationship between the carer and the person being cared for and to the type of care provided. At the same time, the age of the person being cared for is closely related to the relationship between the carer and the cared-for person. Any relationship between service receipt and where care is received or age may, therefore, be determined by any one or a combination of those other intervening variables, rather than the single independent variable under scrutiny.

Where this problem cannot be tackled by quasi-experimental methods, such as the creation of matched groups, as in Chapter Three, this sort of analytical problem inevitably leads the researcher to multi-variate analysis. In this a number of variables can be controlled for simultaneously in an attempt to reveal the true strength of association, if any, between the dependent variable (in this case, service receipt) and independent variables of interest.

Because of the very strong links between the age of the cared-for person, his or her relationship to the carer, and whether or not he/she lived in the same household as the carer, a 'caring relationship' variable which combined all this information was constructed. After a number of experimental stages the following categories were devised:

- relative, aged under 16, in the same household

- relative, aged 16–74, in the same household

- relative, aged 75+, in the same household

- relative, aged 16–74, in a different household

- relative, aged 75+, in a different household

- non-relative, aged 16–74, in a different household

- non-relative, aged 75+, in a different household

- other (includes all non-relatives in the same household, all dependent children not in the same household).

The numbers in each category are shown in Table 5.1.

Table 5.1   Numbers and percentages in each category of caring relationship

Caring relationship	All carers		Main carers only*	
	n	%	n	%
relative, under 16, same hh	77	3	49	3
relative, 16–74, same hh	445	15	364	20
relative, 75+, same hh	235	8	188	10
relative, 16–74, different hh	736	24	411	23
relative, 75+, different hh	881	29	515	28
non-relative, 16-74,different hh	228	8	105	6
non-relative, 75+, different hh	394	13	175	10
other	18	1	14	1
Total	3,014	100	1,821	100

* those with sole, main or joint main responsibility.

Missing from the 1985 GHS data, for most of the people being cared for, is any indication of their level of need for help from others. As we discussed in Chapter Four, the approach adopted here will be to ask whether services appear to discriminate between carers providing similar types and levels of care and, if so, on what basis. In order to do this, both the type of care provided, and the caring relationship, are used in the analysis that follows. The caring categories were further condensed for this stage of the analysis into personal (*personal and physical care* and *personal not physical care*), physical (*physical not personal care*), and other (*other practical help, practical help only* and *other help*). The analysis is also restricted to those carers who carried sole, main or joint main responsibility for the person being cared for. To ease interpretation of findings all services are considered separately in this chapter rather than grouped as in the previous chapter.

The analysis
Logit analysis was used to investigate the relationships between service receipt and other variables. This process allows a num-

ber of dependent variables to be controlled for simultaneously. By designating a comparison category, one can then calculate the relative probability of service receipt for other sub-groups, all other things being equal. Thus, for example, one can calculate the relative probability of a female carer looking after someone who receives a service compared to a male carer, while holding constant the nature of the relationship and the type of care provided.[12]

The analysis in this chapter is in four sections. In the first section, service receipt is the dependent variable and the influence of the caring relationship (outlined above) and the type of care provided arc investigated. In the second section, the sex of the carer is added to the analysis. In the third section, the influence of whether or not the carer was the same sex as the cared-for person on the receipt of selected services is investigated. In the fourth section we attempt to tease out the 'living alone' effect referred to in Chapter Four. Finally, labour market participation and service receipt are considered.

The caring relationship and type of care

In this section we look at receipt of a range of services and how this varied, first by the caring relationship with the type of care provided held constant, and secondly by the type of care provided with the caring relationship held constant. In both cases the results are presented as relative probabilities with a predetermined category for comparison, which has a designated 'probability' of 1.00.

For the caring relationship variable the comparison category is specified as relatives aged 75 and over, living in another household. For the type of care the comparison category is specified as people receiving personal care from the carer. In one or two instances service receipt in some categories was so low, or even non-existent, that it was impossible to compute meaningful probabilities.

---

12 All the analyses presented here are based on 'adequate' models of the relationship between the dependent and independent variables. That is, the variables included in the analysis adequately account for most of the variation observed and the models generate X^2 values which indicate that there are no remaining significant differences to be explained.

Visits from a doctor

Table 5.2 shows the relative probability of the cared-for person's having received regular visits (at least once a month) from a doctor, first by the type of care received and then by the type of caring relationship.

Table 5.2   Relative probability of receiving visits from a doctor

	Relative probability
Type of care: personal	1.00
physical	0.89
other	0.40+
Caring relationship:	
relative, under 16, same hh	0.10+
relative, 16–74, same hh	0.35+
relative, 75+, same hh	0.51+
relative, 16–74, different hh	0.88
relative, 75+, different hh	1.00
non-relative, 16–74, different hh	1.33
non-relative, 75+, different hh	2.11+
other	0.22

+ statistically different from comparison category

The table suggests that visits from a doctor varied substantially with the type of care provided, when the nature of the caring relationship was controlled for.

If we assume that among main carers, as here, type of care provided is a proxy for level of dependence, Table 5.2 suggests that doctors' visits are, generally speaking, targeted at the most disabled or frail individuals. This makes the other finding outlined all the more worrying. Here we see that if type of care is controlled for, doctors are less likely to be visiting those who are cared for by relatives and far less likely to be visiting those who live with the relatives who care for them.

Visits from a community or district nurse

Table 5.3 shows that regular visits from a community or district nurse were also, relatively speaking, well targeted. Those receiving personal or physical care from their informal carers were far more likely to be receiving such visits than were those receiving less intense forms of care.

Table 5.3   Relative probability of receiving visits from
a community or district nurse

	Relative probability
Type of care: personal	1.00
physical	0.76
other	0.20+
Caring relationship:	
relative, under 16, same hh	0.29+
relative, 16–74, same hh	0.37+
relative, 75+, same hh	0.51+
relative, 16–74, different hh	0.55+
relative, 75+, different hh	1.00
non-relative, 16–74, different hh	1.78
non-relative, 75+, different hh	1.44
other	0.55

+ statistically different from comparison category

The variation in service receipt by caring relationship, once type of care is controlled for, is not as extreme as with doctors' visits but follows broadly the same pattern. Those being cared for by relatives were less likely to be seeing a nurse than those being cared for by non-relatives, and those being cared for by relatives in the same household were the least likely of all to be receiving visits. Variation by age of the cared-for person was also rather less obvious with visits from a nurse than it was with doctors.

Visits from a health visitor

The health visitors' role is one traditionally associated with young children although they can, and do, assume responsibility for older people also. Table 5.4 reflects both these factors. Young children in the same household were over twice as likely as very elderly relatives living elsewhere (the comparison category) to be receiving regular visits from a health visitor, although, because of the small numbers involved, this difference does not reach statistical significance. All other groups, except very elderly non-relatives living elsewhere, were substantially less likely to receive visits.

These findings suggest a degree of involvement with older people, but only those being cared for by someone from a different household. Among other groups the probability of seeing a health visitor is approximately the same. In sum, age appears to be a more important influence on health visitor activity than other aspects of the caring relationship. As far as type of care is concerned, health visitors were almost equally likely to be visiting those who received personal or physical care, but half as likely to be visiting someone who received a less intense type of care.

Table 5.4   Relative probability of receiving visits from a health visitor

	Relative probability
Type of care: personal	1.00
physical	0.94
other	0.50+
Caring relationship:	
relative, under 16, same hh	2.26
relative, 16–74, same hh	0.31+
relative, 75+, same hh	0.29+
relative, 16–74, different hh	0.37+
relative, 75+, different hh	1.00
non-relative, 16–74, different hh	0.36+
non-relative, 75+, different hh	0.93
other	*

* not calculable
+ statistically different from comparison category

Visits from a social worker

Variation in the relative probability of receiving regular visits from a social worker was more pronounced than with other services (Table 5.5). This was the case both with the type of care received and with the caring relationship.

People receiving physical care or *other* forms of care were substantially less likely to be seeing a social worker than those receiving personal care. This suggests a close focus of service provision on those who are the most disabled. However, even when this was taken into account, there was still very large variation between different caring relationships.

Those being cared for by non-relatives were far more likely to see a social worker regularly than were those cared for by relatives, regardless of whether or not they were in the same household as the carer. Those being cared for by relatives in the same household had a particularly low relative probability of seeing a social worker. Given that disability is, to some degree, controlled for here, these figures suggest a very high level of discrimination against certain caring situations.

Table 5.5   Relative probability of receiving visits from a social worker

	Relative probability
Type of care: personal	1.00
physical	0.44
other	0.35+
Caring relationship:	
relative, under 16, same hh	0.26
relative, 16–74, same hh	0.59
relative, 75+, same hh	0.30+
relative, 16–74, different hh	1.11
relative, 75+, different hh	1.00
non-relative, 16–74, different hh	4.52+
non-relative, 75+, different hh	2.46+
other	*

* not calculable
+ statistically different from comparison category

Visits from a home help

There is a substantial literature on the home help service, much of which suggests that it is poorly targeted (that is, it does not go always to those who need it most) and that it discriminates against certain types of household (Bebbington and Davies, 1983, 1993; Arber et al., 1988).

Table 5.6 shows that the likelihood of receiving home help is similar for those who receive personal care and those who receive physical care. Indeed, the relative probability of receiving help was marginally higher among those getting *physical* rather than *personal* care. People who have help with physical care (for example, getting in and out of bed, and up and down stairs) are probably likely to need help with domestic activities also and, therefore, to have a need for the home help service. However, it seems likely that people receiving personal care will also need help with physical and domestic activities. Given that providing personal care is more demanding for carers (see Chapter Two) one might have hoped to see this sub-group with a *greater* relative probability of receiving home help than those providing physical care.

People caring for dependent children in the same household and those in the 'other' category were so unlikely to be receiving the home help service that it was impossible to calculate relative probabilities for them. Among the other groups quite clear differences emerged. Elderly non-relatives in a different household were almost twice as likely to have a home help as elderly relatives in a different household. Adults between the ages of 16 and 74 were less likely than the comparison category to be receiving home help but, here again, being cared for by someone who was not a relative and living in a different household enhanced the likelihood of receiving help. Those least likely to be receiving home help were very elderly people being cared for by relatives in the same household. This group was about eight times less likely to receive the service than very elderly relatives living outside the carer's household.

Table 5.6 Relative probability of receiving visits from a home help

	Relative probability
Type of care: personal	1.00
physical	1.08
other	0.48+
Caring relationship:	
relative, under 16, same hh	*
relative, 16–74, same hh	0.18+
relative, 75+, same hh	0.13+
relative, 16–74, different hh	0.39+
relative, 75+, different hh	1.00
non-relative, 16–74, different hh	0.69
non-relative, 75+, different hh	1.91+
other	*

* not calculable
+ statistically different from comparison category

Given that the type of care received is controlled for in the analysis, these figures suggest an enduring discrimination in home help service provision in favour of people living without resident carers and against those being helped by relatives.

Meals-on-wheels service

The meals-on-wheels service is another service which substitutes for domestic activity and one which previous research has suggested is distributed in a highly discriminatory way (Arber *et al.*, 1988).

Table 5.7   Relative probability of receiving visits from a meals-on-wheels service

	Relative probability
Type of care: personal	1.00
physical	0.90
other	0.62
Caring relationship:	
relative, under 16, same hh	*
relative, 16-74, same hh	0.09+
relative, 75+, same hh	*
relative, 16–74, different hh	0.30+
relative, 75+, different hh	1.00
non-relative, 16–74, different hh	1.59
non-relative, 75+, different hh	1.84+
other	0.81

* not calculable
+ statistically different from comparison category

Of all the services considered so far, meals-on-wheels appears to be the least well-targeted, as far as type of care received is concerned (Table 5.7). Those receiving physical care were almost as likely as those receiving personal care to be getting meals. However, those receiving 'other' forms of care were not very much less likely to be receiving meals than either of these other groups.

By contrast, there was substantial variation in receipt between different sorts of caring relationships. Relatives under 16 living in the same household, and those aged 75 and over living in the same household were so unlikely to be receiving meals-on-wheels that relative probabilities could not be calculated for them. Relatives aged 16–74 were also unlikely to be receiving

meals, particularly those who were living in a different household.

Here, again, we find a service which is very unlikely to be supporting individuals who live in the same household as the person caring for them, regardless of their age or the type of care
they receive, and which is more likely to support those cared for
by non-relatives rather than by relatives, even when they do
live in a different household.

Other visitors

Information about visits from other services such as chiropodists, voluntary workers, housing wardens (in sheltered
housing) and any other service was collected in the GHS.
However, housing wardens were making visits almost exclu-
sively to elderly people living somewhere different from the
carer and are therefore excluded from the analysis reported here.
Because of the very small numbers of individuals receiving visits from any of the other services a composite variable was constructed but, even so, only seven per cent of cases had any contact.

Table 5.8   Relative probability of receiving visits from any
other service

	Relative probability
Type of care: personal	1.00
physical	0.62
other	0.41+
Caring relationship:	
relative, under 16, same hh	0.92
relative, 16–74, same hh	0.22+
relative, 75+, same hh	0.27+
relative, 16–74, different hh	0.53+
relative, 75+, different hh	1.00
non-relative, 16–74, different hh	0.39
non-relative, 75+, different hh	0.92
other	*

* not calculable
+ statistically different from comparison category

Table 5.8 shows that receipt of any other service varied with the
type of care received but that, even when this was controlled for,
people in some caring relationship categories were more likely
to be having visits than others.

In contrast to most other services we have looked at, relatives under the age of 16 were almost as likely as those in the comparison category to have received visits from these other services. Non-relatives aged 75 and over who lived elsewhere were also almost as likely to be receiving other services. Overall, there was little evidence of systematic variation related to the age of the person being cared for, or to whether or not s/he was a relative of the carer. This no doubt reflects the diverse nature of services included in this 'other' category.

Any service receipt

Finally in this section which considers the effects of the type of care provided and of the type of caring relationship, we look at the probability of receiving *any* services. Even though this analysis has been restricted to main carers, where the impact of caring is greatest, well under half (39 per cent) of the individuals being cared-for received regular visits from any of the professionals or services considered.

Table 5.9 shows variation of provision related to the type of care provided and, as before, controlling for the caring relationship. Given what has been revealed in previous sections it is not surprising to find that those who receive physical care are somewhat less likely to be receiving any visits than those who receive personal care. Those receiving other types of care are significantly less likely to be receiving any visits.

Table 5.9   Relative probability of receiving any visits

	Relative probability
Type of care: personal	1.00
physical	0.83
other	0.33+
Caring relationship:	
relative, under 16, same hh	0.22+
relative, 16–74, same hh	0.22+
relative, 75+, same hh	0.31+
relative, 16–74, different hh	0.50+
relative, 75+, different hh	1.00
non-relative, 16–74, different hh	0.94
non-relative, 75+, different hh	1.90+
other	0.18+

+ statistically different from comparison category

When type of care is controlled for, a significant pattern of service receipt emerges. Those being cared for by relatives are less likely than those cared for by non-relatives to be receiving any services, and those who live with the caring relative are particularly likely to be poorly served. Service receipt also varies somewhat with age, very elderly people being more likely to receive services than those in younger age groups. As a consequence of all these factors very elderly, non-relatives who live in a different household are almost nine times as likely to receive any services than young children related to and living in the same household as their carer, while very elderly relatives living in a different household are three times as likely to receive services as those living in the same household.

Comparisons across services

With the exception of the meals-on-wheels service, all the services considered appear to be relatively well targeted in relation to the likely level of disability of the person being cared for. However, we have seen very substantial variation in service receipt across different caring relationships, regardless of level of disability. In this sub-section the information about all the services covered is brought together in order to examine whether any systematic differences between them are observable. This also provides an opportunity to look at levels of substitutability in different services.

Table 5.10 shows, as expected, that those being cared for by relatives in the same household are, across the board, less likely to be receiving services than other sub-groups. The only exception here is in relation to visits from a health visitor, which go more often to young children.

However, some services appear to discriminate against some categories of caring relationship even more than others. Thus, for example, the relative probability of receiving a home help service, compared to the comparison category (relative aged 75+ in a different household), is 0.13 for those aged 75 and over who are looked after by a relation in the same household. By contrast the relative probability of people in this group having regular visits from a doctor or from a community nurse is 0.51.

Broadly speaking, the findings presented in Table 5.10 support the suggestions made in earlier research that some form of 'hierarchy' of substitution exists; carers in the same household are apparently less likely to provide nursing or medical care

Table 5.10 Relative probability of receiving a range of services by caring relationship, controlling for type of care

Caring relationship	Relative probability of receiving a service from							
	Doctor	Community nurse	Health visitor	Social worker	Home help	Meals-on-wheels	Other	Any service
relative, under 16, same hh	0.10+	0.29+	2.26	0.26	*	*	0.92	0.22+
relative, 16–74, same hh	0.35+	0.37+	0.31+	0.59	0.18+	0.09+	0.22+	0.22+
relative, 75+, same hh	0.51+	0.51+	0.29+	0.30+	0.13–	*	0.27+	0.31+
relative, 16–74, different hh	0.88	0.55+	0.37+	1.11	0.39+	0.30+	0.53+	0.50+
relative, 75+, different hh	1.00	1.00	1.00	1.00	1.00	1.00	1.00	1.00
non-relative, 16–74, different hh	1.33	1.78	0.36+	4.52+	0.69	1.59	0.39	0.94
non-relative, 75+, different hh	2.11+	1.44	0.93	2.46+	1.91+	1.84+	0.92	1.90+
other	0.22	0.55	*	*	*	0.81	*	0.18+

* not calculable
+ statistically different from comparison category

than to cook or do housework for the cared-for person (Parker, 1990; Arber et al., 1988).

The services also varied in the *spread* of relative probabilities. For example, those most likely to be receiving regular visits from a doctor were 21 times more likely to be doing so than those least likely. For community nursing visits and other services this factor was 5, for health visitors 7, for the home help service 11, for social work 17, for the meals-on-wheels service 21, and for other services 5. This suggests that some services distinguish between different categories of caring relationship much more sharply than do others, community nursing and 'other' services apparently being least influenced by characteristics of the caring relationship and doctors and the meals-on-wheels service most influenced.

Sex of the carer

Evidence about whether or not service providers are more likely to help male informal carers than female informal carers has, until recently, depended on relatively small-scale research. Some of the first research in this area suggested that home help services were provided more often when sons and husbands were the main carers than when daughters and wives were (Hunt, 1978; Bristow, 1981; Charlesworth et al., 1983; Bebbington and Davies, 1983; Wright, 1985), regardless of the degree of disability of the cared-for person.

More recently, as outlined in the introduction, Arber and her colleagues have suggested that it is not the sex of the carer, as such, which influences service provision to elderly people but rather the complex inter-relationship of household composition, sex of the carer, sex of the cared-for person, the carer's employment status and the substitutability of the service itself. Thus, when the degree of the elderly person's disability was controlled for, lone female carers were found to receive no less support than lone male carers. However, *married* women carers under 65 received the lowest levels of domestic and personal health care support. This research also showed the substantial extent to which elderly couples supported one another without service intervention (Arber et al., 1988; Arber and Gilbert, 1989).

The 1985 GHS, of course, covered all ages of cared-for people, not just older ones. Was there any evidence here to suggest that service provision discriminated in some way against female carers?

In order to test this hypothesis the analysis reported in the previous section was re-run, but with sex of the carer as an additional variable. In other words, the analysis explored whether or not men were more likely to get services than women, controlling both for the type of care provided and the caring relationship. As before, the analysis was confined to main carers so that the type of care provided could act as a broad proxy for the degree of disability of the cared-for person.

Adding sex to the analysis made little difference to the relative probability of receiving services in different caring relationships or when different types of care were provided. Further, as Table 5.11 shows, when caring relationship and type of care were controlled for, there was little difference in service receipt between those who had female carers and those who had male carers.

Table 5.11   Relative probability of receiving a range of services by sex of carer, controlling for caring relationship and type of care

Type of service	Relative probability of receiving service (comparison category = male)	
	Male carer	Female carer
Doctor	1.00	1.03
Community nurse	1.00	1.14
Health visitor	1.00	0.84
Social worker	1.00	0.93
Home help	1.00	0.78
Meals-on-wheels	1.00	0.88
Other service	1.00	1.11
Any service	1.00	0.92

Female carers were marginally less likely to be looking after people who received regular visits from a health visitor, a social worker, a home help or the meals-on-wheels service, but these differences were not statistically significant. Conversely, female carers were marginally more likely to be looking after those who had regular visits from a doctor, community nurse or some other service. Again however these differences were not large enough to be statistically significant.

When sex of the carer and his/her marital status were considered together, some of these patterns were strengthened (Table 5.12).

Table 5.12   Relative probability of receiving a range of
services by sex and marital status of carer, controlling
for caring relationship and type of care

| | Relative probability of receiving service if carer is: | | | |
Type of service	Male married	Female married	Male not married	Female not married
Doctor	1.00	0.91	0.91	1.33
Community nurse	1.00	1.14	1.13	1.24
Health visitor	1.00	0.87	1.93	1.28
Social worker	1.00	0.70	0.56	1.24
Home help	1.00	0.79	1.44	0.90
Meals-on-wheels	1.00	0.77	0.87	0.76
Other service	1.00	1.10	0.38	0.63
Any service	1.00	0.92	1.27	1.08

Here we can see that the relative probability of a male carer who
is not married, looking after someone who receives a home
help service is nearly two-thirds higher than that of a female
carer who is not married.

By contrast, female carers who are not married are more likely
than male, not married carers to be looking after someone who
sees a social worker regularly. Married women are less likely
than married men to be caring for someone who receives regular visits from a doctor, health visitor, social worker, home help
or meals-on-wheels service. By contrast the people married
women care for are more likely to be seeing a community nurse
regularly.

Interestingly, the meals-on-wheels service shows the least variation by sex/marital status of the carer. However, alone of any of
the services covered here, this is the one which those cared for
by married male carers are *most* likely to be getting.

Although these patterns are interesting, and in line with some
of what might be expected from earlier research on carers and
services, it should be pointed out that none of the relative probabilities displayed in Table 5.12 is statistically different from 1.00
(that is, the comparison category).

Cross-sex caring

Finally in this section we examine whether cross-sex caring, of itself, influences service receipt. The analysis was run again, this time with a cross-sex variable and controlling for the caring relationship and the type of care provided. As before the analysis was confined to main carers. Table 5.13 shows the results of this analysis for a range of services.

Table 5.13   Relative probability of receiving a range of services by sex of carer and cared-for person, controlling for caring relationship and type of care provided

Type of service	Relative probability of receiving service (comparison category = female/female)			
	Sex of carer/sex of cared-for person			
	Male/ male	Male/ female	Female/ male	Female/ female
Doctor	0.90	0.91	0.80	1.00
Community nurse	0.92	0.78	0.81	1.00
Health visitor	1.11	0.92	0.51	1.00
Social worker	0.69	1.04	0.66	1.00
Home help	1.33	1.31	0.98	1.00
Meals-on-wheels	2.05+	1.20	1.43	1.00
Other service	0.41+	0.89	0.54+	1.00
Any service	1.11	1.02	0.86	1.00

+ statistically different from comparison category

Overall, men being cared for by women had a lower relative probability of receiving any services, but there was variation service by service. Thus men cared for by women were the group least likely to be receiving regular visits from a doctor, health visitor, social worker or a home help. When women were being cared for by men there was a greater relative probability of regular visits from a social worker. However, none of these differences was statistically significant.

The relative probability of men who were cared for by men receiving meals-on-wheels was much higher than for any other group. Home help services were more likely to be going to women being cared for by men than they were to men being cared for by women. This suggests, in line with previous research, that home help services serve to replace disabled women's domestic labour rather than to support women who have caring responsibilities. Further, in this instance, it does seem to be the sex of the carer which is more influential than whether or not he or she is a different sex from the person being helped.

The data presented in this section neither disprove nor prove previous arguments about bias in service provision against those who have female carers. Most of the variation is accounted for by characteristics of the caring relationship (age of the cared-for person, whether or not a relative of the carer, whether or not living in the same household) and the type of care provided (and, thereby, to a degree, the level of disability of the cared-for person).

Adding sex to the analysis does suggest that those with female carers are marginally less likely to get any services, particularly when those female carers are married. However, there is variation between different sorts of services, and few of the differences revealed are large enough to reach statistical significance. Neither is there any suggestion of systematic bias in service provision to those being helped by carers of the opposite sex.

Living alone

We have already seen that those who live in the same household as the person who cares for them are systematically less likely to be receiving services than those whose carer lives elsewhere, regardless of their level of disability. To what extent is this accounted for by services going preferentially to those who live alone who, by definition, have no carer living with them?

In order to explore this issue the following analysis has been restricted to those living in a different household from their main carer.[13] Table 5.14 shows that people living with others, even when their main carer lived elsewhere, were *more* likely to get some type of regular service. However, there was a degree of variation across the different services.

Those living with others were significantly more likely to receive regular visits from a doctor or community nurse, even when the caring relationship and type of care provided were controlled for. Further, health visitors, social workers, meals-

---

[13] This includes a small proportion (21 per cent) whose carer stated that she/he shared responsibility with another carer. It is possible that this other carer lived in the cared-for person's household but there is no way which this can be ascertained from the GHS data.

on-wheels and other services were somewhat more likely to go to those living with others.

Table 5.14   Relative probability of receiving a range of services by whether or not cared-for person lives alone, controlling for caring relationship and type of care provided (all with main carers in different household)

Type of service	Relative probability of receiving services (comparison category = living alone)	
	Living alone	Living with others
Doctor	1.00	1.70+
Community nurse	1.00	1.76+
Health visitor	1.00	1.22
Social worker	1.00	1.42
Home help	1.00	0.75
Meals-on-wheels	1.00	1.10
Other	1.00	1.23
Any service	1.00	1.30+

+ statistically different from comparison category

There may be two possible explanations for this pattern of service receipt. First, it may be that others in the household alert service providers more often to the need for some form of input. Those who live alone, even though they have carers, do not have the continual surveillance that might trigger such demands. A second possibility is that there is something which makes service providers more alert to the cared-for person's needs when they live with others. For example, others in the household may themselves be frail or ill, thus prompting a higher degree of service provision for the cared-for person. Unfortunately, the GHS gives us no information about others in the household of those who do not live with the carer, therefore this possibility cannot be tested.

The only service which those living with others were less likely to be getting than those living alone was the home help service. This finding underlines yet again the very clear nature of the home help service which is to substitute for non-available 'others', rather than to support available others, whether they are carers or not.

Service receipt and employment status

Finally, in this chapter, we examine the impact of service receipt, if any, on carers' labour market participation. Does service receipt allow carers to take paid work or is it at such a low level overall that it makes little difference?

As in previous sections of this chapter we examine receipt of services by controlling for the variable of interest (whether or not carers were in paid work) as well as the type of care provided and the nature of the relationship between the carer and the person being helped. The analysis here was restricted to those under pensionable age (65 years for men and 60 for women) and was carried out separately for men and women.

Table 5.15   Relative probability of female carers (<60) receiving a range of services by whether or not carer was in paid work, controlling for caring relationship and type of care provided

Type of service	Relative probability of receiving services (comparison category = in paid work)	
	In paid work	Not in paid work
Doctor	1.00	1.27
Community nurse	1.00	1.37
Health visitor	1.00	1.42
Social worker	1.00	2.49+
Home help	1.00	1.09
Meals-on-wheels	1.00	1.00
Other	1.00	0.70
Any service	1.00	1.37+

+ statistically different from comparison category

Table 5.15 shows that, overall, female carers not in paid work were significantly more likely to be receiving services than carers in paid work. This was true of all specific services except meals-on-wheels and 'other', but the difference was significant only for social work.

The pattern among male carers was much more variable (Table 5.16). Overall, those not in paid work were only fractionally more likely than those in paid work to be receiving any service, but this disguises considerable differences between particular services. People cared for by men not in paid work, for example, were substantially more likely to be receiving visits from a community nurse. By contrast, they were much less likely to be receiving visits from a doctor, a health visitor or 'other' services. There is no suggestion, then, that services act to enable either male or female carers to participate in the labour market. Indeed, given that the type of care being provided and the relationship between the carer and cared-for person were controlled for, it appears that service provision discriminates against those whose carers are in paid work. However, few of the relationships outlined here are sufficiently strong to allow firm conclusions to be drawn. Further, in the absence of information about the reasons why carers were not in paid work it is difficult even to speculate about cause and effect in relation to the role of services.

Table 5.16   Relative probability of male carers (<65) receiving a range of services by whether or not carer was in paid work, controlling for caring relationship and type of care provided

	Relative probability of receiving services (comparison category = in paid work)	
Type of service	In paid work	Not in paid work
Doctor	1.00	0.54
Community nurse	1.00	2.04+
Health visitor	1.00	0.35
Social worker	1.00	1.73
Home help	1.00	0.97
Meals-on-wheels	1.00	1.38
Other	1.00	0.50
Any service	1.00	1.04

+ statistically different from comparison category

Conclusion

The analysis presented here suggests that while services are usually well targeted towards those cared-for people who might have most need of them, those who have resident carers or who are supported by relatives are substantially under-represented.

However, there is evidence that some form of hierarchy of service substitution exists which is in line with that suggested in earlier research. Further, some services appear to be much more 'influenced' than others by where and with whom cared-for people were living.

There is little evidence to suggest the systematic discrimination against female carers, *per se*, that earlier research has identified. Neither was there any substantial evidence of differential service response to cross-sex caring relationships.

The finding that those without resident carers who also live alone are less likely to receive any service (with the exception of the home help service) raises questions about whether those without resident carers do get more services because service providers are more likely to target those who live alone. This leaves us with the very firm conclusion that, all other relevant things being equal, service provision overall is biased against both those who have resident carers, and those whose carers are related to them.

Counting on carers

The capacity of the 'community', and particularly family members, to provide help and assistance to disabled and older people is arguably more important now than at any other time in recent history. As we outlined in Chapter One, demographic, social, economic and policy changes have combined to increase both the numbers and proportions of people living in the community who require assistance from others to carry out everyday activities.

The increasing emphasis on the role of carers in delivering the objectives of community care policy makes the 1985 GHS information all the more valuable. The survey provided, for the first time, a comprehensive, nationally representative picture of informal caring activity in Great Britain. Secondary analysis of data from the survey has allowed more detailed insight into the range and extent of caring activity in the population. This will enable both policy makers and practitioners to make more accurate estimates of the numbers of heavily involved carers and to recognise them more easily. Further, the analysis has confirmed the effects on heavily involved carers' social and economic circumstances that earlier, small-scale research suggested. We have also shown that health and social care services rarely serve to support heavily involved carers when they are close relatives of the person they are assisting and/or when they live in the same household.

However, as valuable as the 1985 data were, there are two major questions which they raise rather than answer.

First, knowing the numbers and proportions of adults who say that they help others in the community on an unpaid basis is not a real guide to the 'need' for informal care. Some disabled and older people live without substantial support from family, friends or neighbours because they receive formal services or because they have packages of support which they have put together themselves. Others may be able to live without help from anyone else because they have housing which is suitable for their needs and have good adaptations and equipment.

Personal support services, for example, may mean that disabled people do not have to rely on family members and friends. Well-designed toilets and bathrooms may reduce the need for carers to help with personal care. Accessible transport systems may mean that disabled people can travel independently. All the factors which can transform an impairment into a disability also tend to transform family members and friends into 'informal carers' (Oliver, 1990; Morris, 1991). Consequently, interventions which reduced disability and 'dependence' would also reduce the numbers of carers. From this perspective, then, an index of the success of community care policies might be a *reduction* in the numbers of carers.

The second question left unanswered by the 1985 GHS data is the extent to which the population of informal carers *is* changing. One of the most frequently expressed anxieties about informal care is that its supply will shrink under the multiple pressures of decreasing family size, changes in women's labour market participation, changing attitudes towards family obligations and so on. Although there has been much speculation about this issue there is little hard evidence to support arguments one way or another. Indeed, only longitudinal studies or large-scale data sets collected at regular intervals *can* satisfactorily address questions of changing supply.

Some questions about caring responsibilities from the 1985 survey were repeated in 1990 (OPCS, 1992). Obviously two points in time do not allow us to come to hard and fast conclusions about the supply of informal care; changes in either direction could represent random variation between the two points in time. A third 'point' of data collection in the future will be needed to confirm or deny apparent trends revealed between 1985 and 1990. However, the repetition of selected questions does allow some speculation about possible change.

Initial analysis of the 1990 data (Parker and Lawton, 1993) gives an initial impression of a slight dilution in the intensity of caring activity; the hours involved are somewhat shorter, a smaller proportion of carers are apparently involved in the heaviest activities, there is less 'main' and more 'joint' responsibility, and there is a reduction in the extent to which carers live in the same household as the person they assist.

This dilution is, however, more apparent than real. The *numbers* of heavily involved carers have undoubtedly increased (from around 1.76m in 1985 to 1.94m in 1990) while the people being helped are generally older and appear somewhat more likely to have mental impairments or mental health problems. Most important, perhaps, is the evidence of a growing divide between more and less heavily involved carers. There is an increased proportion of older carers and women providing the most intensive forms of help to a generally older group of people, often their parents or parents-in-law or spouse. By contrast, those who were identified in our analysis of the 1985 survey as 'helpers' are providing relatively few hours of practical or 'other' assistance to people who, by and large, live in a different household.

These shifts at both ends of the spectrum of caring activity have clear service implications, pointing to the continued need to encourage low-level input from 'helpers' while providing real support to, or perhaps even taking over from, those who are most heavily involved, if this is what they and the person they assist wish. The extent to which the new community care arrangements can deliver these ends remains to be seen. Small-scale, locally-based evaluation can give some idea of change, but it will require the collection of national data at another point in the near future to provide convincing evidence.

From caring relationships to carers

The development of the caring typology, as outlined in Chapter Two, was based on instances of caring relationships. Because some carers were looking after more than one person the number of carers is actually smaller than the number of caring relationships. This presents some potential problems for any analysis which attempts to examine the characteristics of carers and their relationship to the cared-for person within each care type, because some carers will appear more than once. A less problematic duplication arises where an individual carer appears more than once in different categories of caring. Table A1.1 shows the numbers of carers helping different numbers of people in each care category.

There are several ways in which the problem of carers looking after more than one person in each caring category might be dealt with. One possibility would be simply to base the analysis only on carers. This, however, presents an un-resolvable difficulty with the analysis. Within the data set, the sex, age or economic activity (to take a few examples) of the carer cannot vary dependent upon whether or not she/he looks after more than one person. However, other variables – such as whether she/he is the main carer, whether the cared-for person lives in the same household or elsewhere, the relationship between the carer and cared-for person – could. Where a variable has the same value for the same carer over different cared-for people, then any analysis based on the carer under-represents the prevalence of this value. Where a variable has a different value for the same carer over different cared-for people then analysis based on the carer becomes uninterpretable.

A second approach would be to select at random one cared-for person for each carer who looks after more than one person and base the analysis only on these cases. The major disadvantage of this approach is that it reduces the number of cases available for analysis, especially for the least intensive categories of care where there is a substantial amount of 'multiple caring' and relatively small numbers of caring relationships.

Table A1.1   Numbers of people being cared for in each caring category

Number of people being cared for	Number of people being cared for					Total number of carers	Total number of dependents
	1	2	3	4	5		
Personal *and* physical care	341	15	–	–	–	356	371
Personal *not* physical care	269	7	–	–	–	276	283
Physical *not* personal care	209	16	–	–	–	225	241
Other practical help	150	29	2	–	3	184	229
Practical help only	1,032	204	13	3	1	1,253	1,496
Other help	317	36	5	2	1	360	412

A third possible solution is to assume that those carers who are looking after one person only are little different from those who are looking after more than one. This could then allow one to base the analysis on caring relationships while assuming that this provides a reasonable approximation to carers. If 'multiple carers' are, however, different from 'single carers' then this approach is untenable because it would over-represent the prevalence of that value of the variable(s) which distinguished between them. In fact, there was little difference between single and multiple carers in the different caring categories in relation to sex, age, marital status or economic activity. Further, there was little difference between them with regard to their relationship to the head of the household in which they lived, the number of persons in their household or the number of people (including children) being cared for who lived with them.

Given the importance of these variables in determining other aspects of individuals' experiences, it seems relatively safe to assume that single and multiple carers are similar enough to allow caring relationships to be used as the basis of analysis and to approximate to carers.

In the text, then, reference is made to *carers* although the analysis is actually based on caring *relationships*.

Features of carers in each category of the typology: Summary

1. Carers providing *personal and physical care* were likely to be:

   women (67 per cent)

   caring for a spouse (34 per cent) or child (13 per cent)

   aged 46 or over (66 per cent)

   married (76 per cent) or single (14 per cent)

   working (35 per cent), keeping house (28 per cent) or retired (25 per cent)

   caring for three years or more (64 per cent) and for 20 hours or more a week (68 per cent)

   a sole (38 per cent) or main (32 per cent) carer

   in the same household as the cared-for person (69 per cent).

2. Carers providing *personal not physical care* were likely to be:

   women (74 per cent)

   caring for a parent (28 per cent), child (19 per cent) or 'other' relative (19 per cent)

   aged 46 or over (60 per cent)

   married (74 per cent) or single (12 per cent)

   working (45 per cent), keeping house (26 per cent) or retired (19 per cent)

   caring for five years or more (52 per cent) and for ten hours or more a week (62 per cent)

   a sole (28 per cent) or main (36 per cent) carer

   equally divided between being in the same household or a different one from the cared-for person.

3. Carers providing *physical not personal care* were likely to be:

   equally divided as between men and women

   caring for a parent (39 per cent) or spouse (16 per cent)

   aged between 26 and 65 (78 per cent)

   married (73 per cent) or single (15 per cent)

working (48 per cent), retired (18 per cent) or keeping house (15 per cent)

caring for under ten years (67 per cent) and for between three and 19 hours a week (59 per cent)

without main responsibility (39 per cent) *or* a main carer (27 per cent) in a different household from the cared-for person (61 per cent).

4. Helpers providing *other practical help* were likely to be:

women (60 per cent)

caring for a parent (36 per cent), friend/neighbour (25 per cent) or parent-in-law (15 per cent)

aged between 26 and 65 (81 per cent)

married (76 per cent) or single (12 per cent)

working (56 per cent), keeping house (19 per cent) or retired (15 per cent)

caring for under ten years (70 per cent) and for under ten hours a week (71 per cent)

without main responsibility (36 per cent) *or* a main carer (33 per cent)

in a different household from the cared-for person (88 per cent).

5. Helpers providing *practical help only* were likely to be:

equally divided as between men and women

caring for friends/neighbours (30 per cent), other relatives (25 per cent) or a parent (23 per cent)

aged between 26 and 65 (67 per cent)

married (69 per cent) or single (17 per cent)

working (46 per cent), retired (24 per cent) or keeping house (14 per cent)

caring for under ten years (71 per cent) and for under five hours a week (71 per cent)

without main responsibility (46 per cent) *or* a sole carer (28 per cent)

in a different household from the cared-for person (88 per cent).

6.   Helpers providing *other help* were likely to be:

women (65 per cent)

caring for friends/neighbours (34 per cent), a parent (26 per cent) or 'other' relatives (18 per cent)

aged between 26 and 65 (74 per cent)

married (73 per cent), single (ten per cent) or widowed (ten per cent)

working (55 per cent), keeping house (18 per cent) or retired (15 per cent)

caring for under five years (57 per cent) and for under five hours a week (68 per cent)

without main responsibility (57 per cent)

in a different household from the cared-for person (84 per cent).

Comparison of carers (n= 2516) and non-carers (n= 15814): unmatched

Table A3.1   Sex of carers and non-carers (unmatched)

	Carer %	Non-carer %
Male	40	47
Female	60	53

$X^2 = 50.8$, df = 1, p<0.001

Table A3.2   Age group of carers and non-carers (unmatched)

Age group	Carer %	Non-carer %
16–25	8	19
26–35	13	20
36–45	21	17
46–55	22	12
56–65	20	14
66–75	12	11
76–85	3	6
86+	4	1

$X^2 = 466.1$ df=7, p<0.001

Table A3.3   Marital status of carers and non-carers (unmatched)

Marital status	Carer %	Non-carer %
Married	74	64
Single	13	21
Widowed	7	10
Divorced	4	4
Separated	2	1

$X^2 = 127.6$, df = 4, p<0.001

Table A3.4   Household size of carers and non-carers (unmatched)

Household size	Carer %	Non-carer %
1	9	14
2	39	32
3	19	21
4+	34	34

$X^2 = 77.4$, df = 3, p<0.001

Table A3.5   Economic status of carers and non-carers (unmatched)

Economic status	Carer %	Non-care %
In paid work	64	70
Seeking work	8	7
Permanently unable to work	4	3
Retired	3	2
Keeping house	18	13
Student	2	5
Other inactive	1	1

$X^2 = 83.3$, df = 6, p<0.001

Table A3.6   Comparison of carers' and non-carers' earnings, incomes, household incomes, per capita incomes and equivalent incomes (unmatched)

	Carer £	Non-carer £	
Personal earnings	42	54	p<0.001
Personal income	67	75	p<0.001
Household income	155	164	p<0.01
Per capita income	61	63	p<0.05
LIS[1] equivalent household income	84	87	p<0.05

[1] Luxembourg Income Scale

Table A3.7   General health in past 12 months of carers and
non-carers (unmatched)

General health	Carer %	Non-carer %
Good	59	64
Fairly good	29	25
Not good	13	11

$X^2 = 29.7$, df = 2, p<0.001

Table A3.8   Longstanding illness or disability of carers and
non-carers (unmatched)

Longstanding illness/disability	Carer %	Non-carer %
Yes	40	34
No	60	66

$X^2 = 39.3$, df = 1, p<0.001

Setting up matched groups

Matching was done initially on the basis of age and sex, the two immutable variables which could not have been influenced by caring. Non-carers were chosen from households where no individual was known to be involved in caring. A stratified random sample of non-carers was selected so that they represented the same age group/sex mixture as the carers.

An additional quasi-matching exercise took place in order to look at the impact of different types of caring and of same-household and different-household caring. As Chapter Two showed, people doing different sorts of caring differed from one another quite considerably. If one assumes that different sorts of caring activity are likely to have differential effects on carers, then it is important to tease these effects out from any more general effect of 'being a carer'.

In order to do this the non-carers were sub-divided into six groups, equal in number to and matching on age group and sex, the six caring category sub-groups of the carers. A similar process was used for same-household and different-household care.

The problem of non-response

Although the GHS aims to carry out individual interviews with all adult (16+) members of its sample households, this is not always achieved. Further, some individuals may choose not to answer particular sections of the questionnaire. Obviously, any analysis which attempts to compare one sub-group within the GHS with another (in this case carers with non-carers) needs to bear both forms of non-response in mind.

A comparison of those for whom there was no information about whether or not they had any caring responsibilities shows that they were different from those for whom there was information. Non-respondents were more likely to be: male; aged 16–25 or 86+; never married; in paid work or unable to work; in poor health; from somewhat larger households (three or more individuals); and not to have received any further education. Some of these variables are, of course, inter-related: old age and poor health, for example, or youth and marital status.

In all, the data on non-respondents suggest a picture of young, single men, still living at home with their parents or, perhaps, with friends. Most would be in paid work but there was also a significant, although small, sub-group who were permanently unable to work. In sum, they seemed a group who, other things being equal, were unlikely to have been carers anyway.

Sources of income and receipt of benefits

Table A5.1 in Appendix 5 compares carers and non-carers overall, as well as on the basis of their sex, caring category, and
whether or not they were in the same household. Only those
sources of income which showed significant differences are
reported. The comparison of caring categories and same or different household care is based on the quasi-matching exercise.
Table A5.2 similarly compares benefits received by carer and
non-carer households.

**Table A5.1 Proportion of carers and matched non-carers
receiving specified type of income: overall, by sex, by care
type, and by whether or not in same household**

(i) Overall

	Carer %	Non-carer %
Earnings	50	53 *
Invalidity benefit	3	2 *
Attendance allowance	2	<1 ***
Other short-term benefit	(1)	(9) *

( ) = number

(ii) Male/Female

	Male		Female	
	Carer	Non-carer	Carer	Non-carer
	%	%	%	%
Earnings	58	64 *		
Supplementary benefit	12	9 **		
Invalidity benefit	6	3 *		
Attendance allowance			2	<1 ***
Other short-term benefit			(1)	(8) *

( ) = number

(iii) Caring category

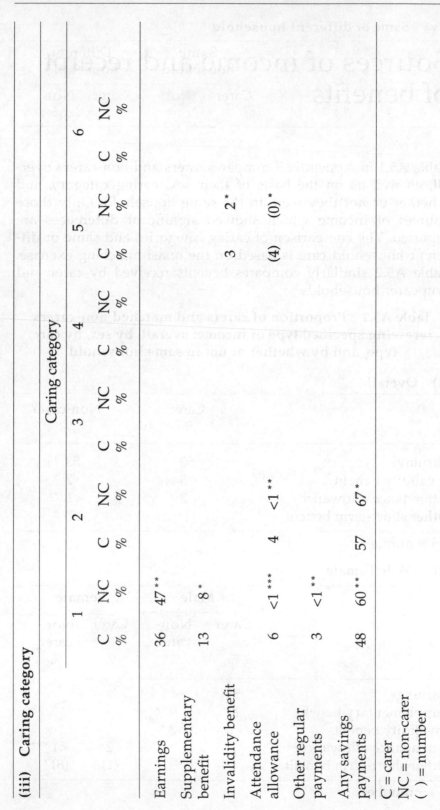

| | Caring category | | | | | | | | | | | |
| | 1 | | 2 | | 3 | | 4 | | 5 | | 6 | |
	C %	NC %	C %	NC %	C %	NC %	C %	NC %	C %	NC %	C %	NC %
Earnings	36	47**										
Supplementary benefit	13	8*										
Invalidity benefit									3	2*		
Attendance allowance	6	<1***	4	<1**					(4)	(0)*		
Other regular payments	3	<1**										
Any savings payments	48	60**	57	67*								

C = carer
NC = non-carer
( ) = number

(iv)   Same or different household

	Same household		Different household	
	Carer	Non-carer	Carer	Non-carer
	%	%	%	%
Earnings	38	46 **		
Supplementary benefit	13	9 *		
Attendance allowance	5	<1 ***		
Any savings	48	58 ***		

X^2 sig at 0.05 level (*), 0.01 level (**), 0.001 level (***)

**Table A5.2   Receipt of benefits by carer and matched
non-carer households: overall, by sex, by care type, and
by whether or not in same household (significant
comparisons only)**

(i)   Overall

	Carer households %	Non-carer households %	
State pension	29	26	*
Supplementary benefit	17	14	**
Sickness benefit	1	<1	**
Invalidity benefit	9	4	***
Disablement benefit	2	<1	***
Attendance allowance	7	<1	***
Mobility allowance	5	1	***
Other short-term	<1	1	*
Other long-term	3	1	***
Any benefit	**76**	**71**	***

(ii)   Sex

	Male		Female	
	Carer %	Non-carer %	Carer %	Non-carer %
State pension	29	24 *		
Supplementary benefit	17	12 **		
Sickness benefit			1	<1 ***
Invalidity benefit	8	4 ***	9	4 ***
Disability benefit	2	<1 ***	1	<1 *
Attendance allowance	7	<1 ***	7	<1 ***
Mobility allowance	6	1 ***	5	1 ***
Other short-term			(2)	(9) *
Other long-term			3	1 ***
Any benefit	**74**	**69** *	**77**	**73** *

(iii)   Caring category

	__ 1 __		__ 2 __		__ 3 __		__ 4 __		__ 5 __		__ 6 __	
	C %	NC %	C %	NC %	C %	NC %	C %	NC %	C %	NC %	C %	NC %
State pension	43	35										–
Supplementary benefit	27	13	21	12								
Invalidity benefit	11	5	14	5	14	5	7	4			9	4
Disability benefit	4	1	4	<1								–
Attendance allowance	28	<1	12	<1	2		2	<1			3	<1
Mobility allowance	16	1	8	2	7	1	3	1				
Other long term					2		2	1			4	1
Any benefit	87	73	80	72	84	69						

(iv)   Same or different household

	Same household		Different household	
	Carer	Non-carer	Carer	Non-carer
	%	%	%	%
State pension	49	35 ***		
Supplementary benefit	25	15 ***		
Sickness benefit	2	6 **		
Invalidity benefit	19	4 ***		
Disability benefit	5	<1 ***		
Attendance allowance	23	<1 ***		
Mobility allowance	16	1 ***		
Other short-term	(0)	(4) *		
Other long-term	6	1 ***		
Any benefit	**90**	**73** ***		

X^2 sig at 0.05 level (*), 0.01 level (**), 0.001 level (***)
( ) = number

References

ALDENDERFER, M.S. and BLASHFIELD, R.K. (1984) *Cluster Analysis*, Beverly Hills: Sage.

ARBER, S. and GILBERT, N. (1989) 'Men: the forgotten carers', *Sociology*, 23, 1, 111–18.

ARBER, S. and GINN, J. (1990) 'The meaning of informal care: gender and the contribution of elderly people', *Ageing and Society*, 10, 4, 429–54.

ARBER, S. and GINN, J. (1991) *Gender and Later Life: A Sociological Analysis of Resources and Constraints*, London: Sage.

ARBER, S. and GINN, J. (1992) 'In sickness and in health: Caregiving, gender and the independence of elderly people' in MARSH, C. and ARBER, S. (eds) *Families and Households: Divisions and Change*, London: Macmillan.

ARBER, S., GILBERT, N. and EVANDROU, M. (1988) 'Gender, household composition and receipt of domiciliary services by the elderly disabled', *Journal of Social Policy*, 17, 2, 153–75.

AYER, S. and ALASZEWSKI, A. (1984) *Community Care and the Mentally Handicapped: Services for Mothers and their Mentally Handicapped Children*, London: Croom Helm.

BALDWIN, S.M. (1985) *The Costs of Caring*, London: Routledge and Kegan Paul.

BALDWIN, S. and PARKER, G. (1989) 'The Griffiths report on community care' in BRENTON, M. and UNGERSON, C. (eds) *Social Policy Review 1988–9*, Harlow: Longman.

BEBBINGTON, A.C. and DAVIES, B. (1983) 'Equity and efficiency in the allocation of personal social services', *Journal of Social Policy*, 12, 3, 309–30.

BEBBINGTON, A.C. and DAVIES, B. (1993) 'Efficient targeting of community care: the case of the home help service', *Journal of Social Policy*, 23, 3, 373–91.

BRADSHAW, J. and LAWTON, D. (1978) 'Tracing the causes of stress in families with handicapped children', *British Journal of Social Work*, 8, 2, 181–92.

BRISTOW, A.K. (1981) *Crossroads Care Attendant Schemes: A Study of their Organisation and Working Practice and of the Families whom they Support*, Association of Crossroads Care Attendants Schemes, Rugby.

BULMER, M. (1987) *The Social Basis of Community Care*, London: Allen & Unwin.

CHARLESWORTH, A., WILKIN, D. and DURIE, A. (1983) *Carers and Services: a Comparison of Men and Women Caring for Dependent Elderly People*, University of Manchester, Departments of Psychiatry and Community Medicine.

DH/DSS/WELSH OFFICE/SCOTTISH OFFICE (1989) *Caring for People: Community Care in the Next Decade and Beyond*, Cm 849, London: HMSO.

DEPARTMENT OF HEALTH AND SOCIAL SECURITY *et al.* (1981) *Growing Older*, Cmnd. 8173, London: HMSO.

EQUAL OPPORTUNITIES COMMISSION (1982) *Caring for the Elderly and Handicapped: Community Care Policies and Women's Lives*, Manchester: EOC.

EVANDROU, M. (1990) *Challenging the Invisibility of Carers: Mapping Informal Care Nationally*, Discussion Paper WSP/49, STICERD, London School of Economics.

FOSTER, K., WILMOT, A. and DOBBS, J. (1990) *General Household Survey 1988*, London: HMSO.

GLENDINNING, C. (1983) *Unshared Care*, London: Routledge and Kegan Paul.

GLENDINNING, C. (1992) *The Costs of Informal Care: Looking Inside the Household*, London: HMSO.

GREEN, H. (1988) *General Household Survey 1985: Informal Carers*, London: HMSO.

GRIFFITHS, R. (1988) *Community Care: An Agenda for Action*, London: HMSO.

HARRIS, A. (1971) *Handicapped and Impaired in Great Britain*, London: HMSO.

HIRST, M.A. (1990) 'Financial independence and social security', *Children and Society*, 4, 1, 70–78.

HOUSE OF COMMONS (1974) *Social security provision for chronically sick and disabled people*, London: House of Commons Paper 276.

HUNT, A. (1978) *The Elderly at Home*, OPCS Social Survey Division, London: HMSO.

ISAACS, B., LIVINGSTON, M. and NEVILLE, Y. (1972) *Survival of the Unfittest: A Study of Geriatric Patients in Glasgow*, London: Routledge & Kegan Paul.

JOSHI, H. (1987) 'The cost of caring' in GLENDINNING, C. and MILLAR, J. (eds) *Women and Poverty*, Brighton: Wheatsheaf Books.

KING'S FUND INFORMAL CARING PROGRAMME (1988) *Action for Carers: A Guide to Multi-Disciplinary Support at Local Level*, London: King's Fund Centre.

KING'S FUND CENTRE FOR HEALTH SERVICES DEVELOPMENT (1992) *Report of a one-day Conference: All Change for Carers?*, London: King's Fund Centre.

LEVIN, E., SINCLAIR, I. and GORBACK, P. (1983) *The Supporters of Confused Elderly People at Home: Extract from the Main Report*, London: National Institute for Social Work Research Unit.

LEWIS, J. and MEREDITH, B. (1988) *Daughters Who Care: Daughters Caring for Mothers at Home*, London: Routledge.

MCLAUGHLIN, E. (1991) *Social Security and Community Care: The Case of the Invalid Care Allowance*, DSS Research Report Series No. 4, London: HMSO.

MORRIS, J. (1991) *Pride Against Prejudice: Transforming Attitudes to Disability*, London: Women's Press.

MORRIS, L. (1987) 'The no-longer working class', *New Society*, 3/4/89, 16–19.

NISSEL, M. and BONNERJEA, L. (1982) *Family care of the Handicapped Elderly: Who Pays?*, London: Policy Studies Institute.

OFFICE OF POPULATION CENSUSES AND SURVEYS SOCIAL SURVEY DIVISION (1989) *General Household Survey 1985* [computer file], Colchester: ESRC Data Archive.

OFFICE OF POPULATION CENSUSES AND SURVEYS SOCIAL SURVEY DIVISION (1992) *General Household Survey 1990*, [computer file], Colchester: ESRC Data Archive.

OLIVER, M.C. (1990) *The Politics of Disablement*, London: Macmillan.

PAHL, J. (1989) *Money and Marriage*, Basingstoke: Macmillan.

PARKER, G. (1985) *With Due Care and Attention: A Review of Research on Informal Care* (1st edition), Occasional Paper No. 2, London: Family Policy Studies Centre.

PARKER, G. (1989) *'The same difference? The Experiences of Men and Women Caring for a Spouse with a Disability or Chronic Illness'*, paper given at Social Policy Association Conference, University of Bath, July 1989.

PARKER, G. (1990a) *With Due Care and Attention: A Review of Research on Informal Care* (2nd edition), London: Family Policy Studies Centre.

PARKER, G. (1990b) 'Whose care? Whose costs? Whose benefit? A critical review of research on case management and informal care', *Ageing and Society*, 10, 459–67.

PARKER, G. (1993) *With This Body: Caring and Disability in Marriage*, Buckingham: Open University Press.

PARKER, G. and LAWTON, D. (1990) *Further Analysis of the 1985 General Household Survey Data on Informal Care. Report 1: A Typology of Caring*, DH 715, Social Policy Research Unit Working Paper, York: Social Policy Research Unit, University of York.

PARKER, G. and LAWTON, D. (1991) *Further Analysis of the 1985 General Household Survey Data on Informal Care. Report 4: Male Carers*, DH 849, Social Policy Research Unit Working Paper, York: Social Policy Research Unit, University of York.

PARKER, G. and LAWTON, D. (1993) *Further Analysis of the 1990 General Household Survey: Report 1*, DH 1061, Social Policy Research Unit Working Paper, York: Social Policy Research Unit, University of York.

PARKER, R. (1981) 'Tending and social policy' in GOLDBERG, E.M. and HATCH, S. (eds) *A New Look at the Personal Social Services*, London: Policy Studies Institute.

PENTOL, A. (1983) 'Cost bearing burdens', *Health and Social Service Journal*, 8/9/83.

QUINE, L. and PAHL, J. (1985) 'Examining the causes of stress in families with severely mentally handicapped children', *British Journal of Social Work*, 15, 501–17.

QURESHI, H. (1986) 'Responses to dependency: reciprocity, affect and power in family relationships' in PHILLIPSON, C., BERNARD, M. and STRANG, P. (eds) *Dependency and Interdependency: Theoretical Perspectives and Policy Alternatives*, Beckenham: Croom Helm.

QURESHI, H. and WALKER, A. (1989) *The Caring Relationship: Elderly People and Their Families*, London: Macmillan.

SIEGEL, S. (1956) *Nonparametric Statistics for the Behavioural Sciences*, Tokyo: McGraw Hill Kogakusha.

SMYTH, M. and ROBUS, N. (1989) *The Financial Circumstances of Families with Disabled Children Living in Private Households*, London: HMSO.

SOCIAL SERVICES INSPECTORATE/SOCIAL WORK SERVICES GROUP (1991) *Care Management Assessment, Summary of Practice Guidance*, London: HMSO.

TWIGG, J. (1989) 'Models of carers: how do social care agencies conceptualise their relationship with informal carers', *Journal of Social Policy*, 18, 1, 53–66.

TWIGG, J. (1992) (ed) *Carers: Research and Practice*, London: HMSO.

TWIGG, J. and ATKIN, K. (1993) *Carers Perceived: Policy and Practice in Informal Care*, Buckingham: Open University Press.

TWIGG, J., ATKIN, K. and PERRING, C. (1990) *Carers and Services: A Review of Research*, London: HMSO.

UNGERSON, C. (1987) *Policy is Personal: Sex, Gender and Informal Care*, London: Tavistock.

WENGER, C. (1984) *The Supportive Network: Coping with Old Age*, London: George Allen & Unwin.

WENGER, C. (1986) 'What do dependency measures measure? Challenging assumptions' in PHILLIPSON, C., BERNARD, M. and STRANG, P. (eds) *Dependency and Interdependency: Theoretical Perspectives and Policy Alternatives*, Beckenham: Croom Helm.

WILSON, G. (1987) *Money in the Family*, Aldershot: Avebury.

WRIGHT, F. (1983) 'Single carers: employment, housework and caring' in Finch, J. and Groves, D. (eds) *A Labour of Love: Women, Work and Caring*, London: Routledge and Kegan Paul.

WRIGHT, F. (1985) *Left to Care Alone*, Gower: Aldershot.

Index

Printed in the United Kingdom for HMSO.
Dd.297145, 1/94, C11, 3396/4, 5673, 269269.